MOVING INTO
RESIDENTIAL CARE

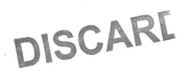

of related interest

Nothing about us, without us!
20 years of dementia advocacy
Christine Bryden
ISBN 978 1 84905 671 7
eISBN 978 1 78450 176 1

People with Dementia Speak Out
Edited by Lucy Whitman
Afterword by Professor Graham Stokes
ISBN 978 1 84905 270 2
eISBN 978 0 85700 552 6

**Introduction to the Psychology
of Ageing for Non-Specialists**
Ian Stuart-Hamilton
ISBN 978 1 84905 363 1
eISBN 978 0 85700 715 5

Positive Communication
Activities to Reduce Isolation and
Improve the Wellbeing of Older Adults
Robin Dynes
ISBN 978 1 78592 181 0
eISBN 978 1 78450 449 6

**A Creative Toolkit for
Communication in Dementia Care**
Karrie Marshall
ISBN 978 1 84905 694 6
eISBN 978 1 78450 206 5

Chair Yoga
Seated Exercises for Health and Wellbeing
Edeltraud Rohnfeld
Illustrated by Edeltraud Rohnfeld
ISBN 978 1 84819 078 8
eISBN 978 0 85701 056 8

MOVING INTO RESIDENTIAL CARE

A Practical Guide for Older People and Their Families

Colleen Doyle
Gail Roberts

Jessica Kingsley *Publishers*
London and Philadelphia

Some case studies throughout have been based on the unpublished booklet 'Caring Moves', written by Gail Roberts and Colleen Doyle for Villa Maria Catholic Homes, copyright © Villa Maria Catholic Homes 2016. Reproduced and adapted with permission.

Figure 5.1 has been reproduced with permission of John Fisher.

Table 6.1 has been adapted with permission of Linda Brownfield.

The box on pages 86–87 has been adapted with permission of APA.

First published in 2018
by Jessica Kingsley Publishers
73 Collier Street
London N1 9BE, UK
and
400 Market Street, Suite 400
Philadelphia, PA 19106, USA

www.jkp.com

Copyright © Colleen Doyle and Gail Roberts 2018

Front cover image source: iStockphoto®.

Library of Congress Cataloging in Publication Data
A CIP catalog record for this book is available from the Library of Congress

British Library Cataloguing in Publication Data
A CIP catalogue record for this book is available from the British Library

ISBN 978 1 78592 189 6
eISBN 978 1 78450 462 5

Printed and bound in Great Britain

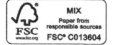

PREFACE AND ACKNOWLEDGEMENTS

This book arose from research conducted while the authors were partnership researchers with a residential care provider in Melbourne, Australia. A booklet, *Caring Moves*, was produced for residents and their families, based on research and interviews conducted during 2015–16 with new residents and family members about their experiences of moving into residential care. Some stories reproduced here (with permission) are from those interviews. This book expands the research and also provides context relevant to people living in the UK, USA, Canada and New Zealand. Recent research on relocation into residential care has been added. We are grateful for the assistance of the residents, family members and staff who agreed to be interviewed in our original study, and acknowledge the support of Villa Maria Catholic Homes, Bridget O'Shannassy and Maria Egan during our work in 2016.

DISCLAIMER AND ADVICE

The views expressed in this book are the authors' alone and provide a general summary only. People should seek professional advice about their specific care needs.

CONTENTS

CHAPTER 1

INTRODUCTION

Moving into a residential care home can be one of the most significant life events of later life. The move to a care home may be anticipated or planned by the older person herself/himself in discussion with family or friends. Often it can be unexpected, precipitated by a personal health crisis that requires hospitalisation, and from there it becomes clear that going back home to live independently is not feasible. For others, a slow decline in health may worry relatives and friends, who then pressure the older person to consider moving into full-time care. Occasionally, a person makes the decision to remain in a care home after they have had an enjoyable respite care experience there. Whatever the circumstances, it can be a stressful experience for the person moving to residential care and for their family and significant others, as they leave behind a familiar life, routine and surroundings.

This book summarises the evidence about what the experience of relocating into a care home feels like and what can help to make the change easier, and shares the stories of some people who have experienced it. There are many different terms used internationally in the area of care (see Appendix 2). For ease of reading, we have adopted the term 'care home' to mean 'care home with nursing' or 'residential care home' or 'nursing home' as there are many terms used internationally for the same thing – communal living for older people with provision of 24 hour nursing and personal care and social care support. We have also used 'family' to mean family or friends or people who are closely associated with the person moving into the care home. We recognise that many people do not have a close association with their biological family, but friends or others close to them form a 'family' for the person.

We describe the experience of moving into a care home and what new residents and their family can do to ease the transition. We also share the experiences of some residents who recently moved into care homes.[1] While these residents were in Australia, there are many commonalities in the provision of care in other countries, and their stories may resonate with older people experiencing similar transitions elsewhere. We interviewed residents, family members and staff about their experiences and asked them about what helped the adjustment process. The stories show a range of experiences and may help future residents and their family members to understand more about the transition process, and what they can do to best cope with the move. The names used in the stories throughout the book are pseudonyms, and some story details have been changed to protect individual residents' anonymity. To illustrate some points, case studies arc also included that are a combination of stories from people we have met in the course of our experience in care.

ORIGINS OF CARE HOMES

Residential care has not always been available. The idea of housing set aside for older people who could no longer live independently

---

[1]   The stories published here are based on a research project using research methods approved by the ACU Human Research Ethics Committee approval number 2015-91E.

came about in the 19th century. Until then, it was expected that older people would be cared for by family if they could no longer care for themselves. For the rich, servants could care for them if family were not available. For those alone and poor, the local 'almshouse' was the only choice. In the UK, the 1834 Poor Law gave 'indoor relief' to sick people living in 'workhouses' where men and women were separated, and people worked for the privilege of living there. In 1861, 50,000 people in the UK were housed in the care of a workhouse medical officer (Peace 2003). Later in the 19th century, reforms started to recognise the rights and care needs of the sick, the unemployed and children. From the 1880s onwards, separate care homes developed to care for people with only a modest income. However, the quality of care was low. By the 1920s, even though there were now substantial numbers of nursing homes (26,000 in England and Wales), a Select Committee on Nursing Homes (Registration) reported on the very dire circumstances in which people were living, and subsequently in 1927 the first registration and inspection process was established.

In other countries, similar health, social and care developments were occurring. In Australia, by the early 1900s, resident rights and care needs were beginning to be considered. The state of nursing homes in Australia was highlighted by the Ronalds (1989) report, and subsequently later governments increasingly regulated the provision of care for older people in these settings. Today residential care provision has evolved to the situation where care that is subsidised by government funding is regulated by government agencies that monitor the quality of care. The monitoring process is complex and often criticised because there continues to be a range of quality of care provided.

TERMS USED FOR 'CARE HOMES' INTERNATIONALLY

Nursing home (UK, USA, Canada, Australia, New Zealand)   Nursing homes provide 24-hour care for individuals, mostly older people, who are not able to live independently. Services include provision of a room, food, personal care, lifestyle or social, recreational activities, and access to emergency care. Staff profiles vary but generally there are some nursing staff, medical staff on call, regular access to primary health care physicians and allied health services. Many residents receive palliative and end-of-life care within the home. Unlike acute hospitals, there is an emphasis on person-centred care, homelike environments and social relationships to ensure quality of life is high.

Convalescent home   Also called sub-acute care or transition care, this is where people can recover from an acute illness or injury for a short time and then return to their own home.

Skilled nursing facility (USA)   A nursing home certified to provide Medicare-funded care. Medicare is the US scheme provided for people over 65 who contributed to social security and Medicare during their working life. Medicaid is a programme to provide health care to people with income below the poverty line.

Care home (UK)   Previously known as residential homes, care homes provide 24-hour care. In order to enter a care home, an individual needs an assessment of their financial and health status from the local council.

Care home with nursing (UK)   Previously known as nursing homes, care homes with nursing provide greater access to nursing care than care homes. Some homes provide both, allowing the resident to age in place as their health deteriorates and they require more assistance.

Rest home (New Zealand)   Also known as aged residential care facilities. Access to these homes is through a specialised assessment team.

Intermediate care facility (USA)   A place to live for people who are elderly, disabled or living with chronic illness. These facilities usually provide less intensive care than an acute hospital or a skilled nursing facility.

Long-term care facility (Canada)   In Canada, long-term care facilities can be private, public or subsidised. The latter two differ only in who owns the facility. Funding, admission and cost to the residents are regulated by the government. Long-term care consists of medical and support services for people who have lost their capacity to live independently.

Board and care home (USA)   Sometimes called residential care homes, these places provide assisted living services. Many are small scale, providing accommodation for less than six people. They still offer 24-hour assistance with staff including licensed health care professionals.

Assisted living facility   These places are used by people with disabilities who may be too young to live in a retirement home; they provide some care but not the 24-hour care provided by a nursing home. The main difference is the level of care the person needs. Assisted living facilities do not usually provide assistance with personal care or nursing/medical care.

Residential home (UK)   Previous term used for places now known as care homes.

Residential aged care facility or residence (Australia)   These facilities provide 24-hour care by a mix of trained nursing and personal care staff. In order to be admitted, residents undergo a comprehensive geriatric assessment. Funding is subsidised by the federal government.

Hospice   Hospices provide palliative or end-of-life care, including medical, nursing and social services. Stays are usually time limited. Some nursing homes provide palliative care at the facility so residents do not need to move near the end of life.

WHAT CAN A CARE HOME PROVIDE?

In modern care homes, we have moved on from the expectation that older people will work in return for their care and board. Care homes have changed dramatically since the early days. Today the care provided in these homes is regulated by the government and quality of care is closely monitored in certain areas, although it can still vary considerably from one home to the next. The characteristic of communal living is still the common denominator for the variety of homes available. The term 'care home' is used for communal living where staff provide assistance to older residents, although the level of assistance varies. In the UK, care home accommodation provides support for older people who are unable to care for themselves. Help with personal care such as washing, dressing and going to the toilet is provided by staff who work at the site, so the residents live there but staff come and go in the same way that acute hospital staff work on site then return to their own homes. Meals and a bed, usually in a private room but not always, are provided. There will usually be shared spaces for social activities, and a shared dining room. Some homes will have a garden that residents can use and there may be a resident pet, or pets may visit from 'pet therapy' services. Some residents are allowed to have visits from their pets brought in by family. Bathrooms may be shared or ensuite. Some care homes offer nursing care as well as care with activities of daily living. For residents with medical needs, some care homes arrange for visits by local family doctors or there may be a medical practice that operates on site during certain days of the week.

In the USA, according to Freedman and Spillman (2014), of people who were Medicare beneficiaries, about 3 million older people were in nursing homes in 2011. People living in nursing homes in the USA have meals provided, assistance with personal care and medication management, laundry and housekeeping and social activities. Transport was available to 85 per cent of these residents, but recreational facilities were only available to about half. According to one survey, the most common unmet need was for getting outside (Freedman and Spillman 2014).

In Australia, residential care homes provide help with day-to-day tasks and health care. Staff help with cleaning, cooking, laundry, personal care and 24-hour nursing care. Each home is different, but the day-to-day routine is expected to be 'person centred', which means that the resident has a say in what routine they would like, for example, in times for rising, showering, meal times, what to eat and so on, although the extent to which this is able to be provided varies from one home to the next. As the living is communal, and staffing is limited by the costs, there are restrictions on how flexible these services can be in reality.

FACTS AND FIGURES ABOUT MOVING INTO CARE

Not everyone will need to move into a care home as they get older; in fact, the majority of older people will not experience living in a care home, although many people will know someone who does. In Australia, the lifetime probability of admission into a care home has been estimated as 20 per cent (Australian Department of Health and Ageing 2011). In the UK, in 2011 there were 9.2 million people in England and Wales aged over 65 (Office for National Statistics 2013). In fact, the number of residential care home places is decreasing relative to the aged population in the UK, in response to consumer preferences to receive care in their own home for as long as possible, and also partly in response to the rising costs of providing residential care. In the UK, according to the Office for National Statistics, the number of people living in care homes has remained the same since 2001, even though the number of people over 65 has been increasing.

In 2011, about 291,000 people over 65 were living in care homes in England and Wales. This only represents 3.2 per cent of the total population over 65, meaning the majority of older people live in the community. For people 75–84 there was actually a decline in the resident care population in the ten years from 2001 to 2011.

Most people living in care homes are over 85 years of age. In the UK in the 2011 census, 10.5 per cent of care home residents were aged 65–74, 30.3 per cent were aged 75–84 and 59.2 per cent were aged over 85 (Office for National Statistics 2014). Most residents are female, partly due to longer life expectancy among women. Among all those 65 and over in the UK, 4.6 per cent of women live in care homes while only 1.9 per cent of men live in care homes.

Most people living in care accommodation have some health problems that make it hard for them to care for themselves independently. When researchers ask people to rate their own health, they find that there is a continuum of experiences among older people, and a surprising number report ill health. Of all the people over 65 in England and Wales, only half reported very good or good health in the 2011 census. Over a third reported bad or very bad health and had health problems or disability that limited their daily activity.

In the USA, the profile of older people living in care homes is similar, with health problems common and a mostly female, older population. While statistics vary according to the study, estimates from Caffrey et al. (2012) showed that nearly 75 per cent of US care home residents were female, about three-quarters of residents received help with self-care and mobility, nearly 45 per cent had dementia and 60 per cent were aged 85 or older. In Canada, the number of older people living in care homes declined between 1981 and 2011. In 2016, 1.2 per cent of Canadians lived in nursing homes (Statistics Canada 2017).

In Australia, residential care and home care are provided to about 273,000 people at any one time, three-quarters of these places being in care homes. Australia has a much smaller population (24 million in 2017) than the UK (65 million in 2017) or USA (326 million in 2017), but the characteristics and use of residential care is broadly similar in all three countries. In Australia, a greater proportion of the aged population live in care homes than in the UK. In 2013–14 in Australia, 7.8 per cent of people over 65 (270,000 people) were in care homes at some point over the financial year. By contrast 83,000 people received care in their own homes during the same year (Australian Institute of Health and Welfare 2017). In Australia, one-third of residential care is provided in rural or remote areas. In 2015, three in five Australians living in care homes were over 85 years of age. A small number of younger people also live in care homes in Australia, but the number and proportion of younger people in care homes has been falling. In 2015, 4 per cent of all Australian care home residents were aged under 65. Two-thirds of people in permanent residential care are women (Australian Institute of Health and Welfare 2017). One in four people in care homes in Australia require a high level of care for activities of daily living, behaviour conditions associated with dementia, and complex health care.

HOW LONG DO PEOPLE LIVE IN CARE HOMES?

The average length of stay in a care home varies from one country to the next. One study in the USA found that half of people moving to care homes died within six months, reflecting their frailty when they moved. The median length of stay was five months (i.e. half of people stayed for a shorter period of time and half stayed for longer), while the average length of stay was 14 months, indicating that some people stay for a much longer period of time (Kelly *et al.* 2010). In the UK, the median length of stay was 20 months, while the median length of stay for people admitted to nursing beds was 12 months and for residential beds it was 27 months (Forder and Fernandez 2011). In Australia, the average length of stay is 2.8 years (Australian Institute of Health and Welfare 2012) while the median length of stay is about two years. Some people use care homes as respite care only, returning to their own homes in between visits to care homes. In Australia, respite care offers short-term care from a few days up to nine weeks for people who need care and a break from living in their own home when their family or main carer goes away. Sometimes people use respite care to try residential care and see whether it suits them when they are thinking about moving into care.

ATTITUDES TO CARE HOMES

The media often portrays care negatively, which may be one reason why the societal view of care continues to be a largely negative one. We rarely hear news of people who are happy to be living in a care home, or of people who are very satisfied with their decision to move. Instead, most media stories are of very negative incidents that occurred in care homes. These stories are sensational, as sensation is interesting and sells newspapers, and can colour our view of what care homes are like to live in. Often, they are unfair to the majority of care providers, who work hard to make life in a care home as pleasant as possible.

While the media promulgate a negative view of care homes, society as a whole also has a dim view of residential care, perhaps stemming from the origin of care homes as places for the poor, and also from the general stigma of being old and frail, known as ageism (prejudice against older people). Studies of attitudes towards care homes have shown that most people do not intend to use a care home if they can avoid it. One study of Japanese-

American older people showed them a series of hypothetical scenarios (McCormick *et al.* 1996). When considering what they would do if they fractured a hip, only 12 per cent of study participants said they would use a care home – about half said they would use paid home care and about a third would recover at home with the help of family or friends. However, when study participants were asked what they would do if they developed dementia, about half indicated that under those circumstances they would use a care home and only 11 per cent intended to rely on family or friends for care. Lack of social support was considered a big factor in the decision about whether or not to use a care home.

CHAPTER 2

MAKING THE DECISION TO MOVE

WHAT DOES HOME MEAN FOR OLDER PEOPLE?

Home is tied to our identity in fundamental ways that are often not noticed until 'home' is taken away. Home is more than bricks and mortar. Researchers have described home as being physical, imaginative and affective in its role as a place of belonging (Brownie, Horstmanshof and Garbutt 2014). In other words, apart from the physical look of the home, there is another layer of what we imagine our home is like in a psychological sense. Our imagined ideal of what a home should be like interacts with the real home to produce feelings about the homeliness or otherwise of our surroundings. So, in a psychological sense, a person's home can truly be viewed as his/her castle, regardless of the reality. This idea of home being more than just the physical reality is also influenced by cultural background, race, physical ability, gender, class and age (Brownie *et al.* 2014). It is this whole psychological perception of home that is disrupted when moving into a care home – not just the physical move, but the added layers of imagined place and emotional ties. Moving to the care home requires rebuilding perceptions of the new 'home', something that is challenging for many people.

A sense of security and shelter may have been built up over many years by someone in the later part of their life. Some older people faced with moving into a care home may be leaving a home that they have lived in for most of their life – a truly daunting prospect. The longer the person has lived in one place, the more challenging the transition to a care home may become. Moving into care may mean that most of the person's possessions have to be disposed of, or at least not taken with the person to their new residence. Researchers have found that 'home' is both a place and has a meaning that develops over time (Johnson and Bibbo 2014). Our self-identity and our life history can be tied up in our possessions and where we live. Home can also be a symbol of what we are, or what our identity consists of. It may represent to the older person that they are healthy, independent and well off. By moving away from this identity, the older person is losing whom they consider themselves to be, so it is understandable that the transition to a care home involves setting up a whole new identity and adjusting to this new view of themselves.

The social life associated with home can also be part of what 'home' means. As people age, home can become a centre of social relationships. Sociologists study social patterns, and as people age their social interactions can be centred more on their home, as older people are visited more than they visit others. When people stay at home more, their personal possessions can take on more importance as their sense of identity is expressed more in their surroundings. When moving to a care home, the individual's identity has to be re-shaped. Understandably, some people continue to identify with their old home and do not consider the care home as a 'real home'.

UNDERSTANDING THE EMOTIONAL ASPECTS OF MOVING INTO CARE

Anyone who has ever moved house understands that it is an unsettling life event. The experience brings mixed feelings.

There is the stress of starting to consider moving and not knowing what the future will hold. Family and friends may have mixed opinions about the wisdom or folly of moving. The financial side of moving will worry many people, especially if they are considering whether the move will impact on their ability to help other family members with financial decisions in the future as well. Not knowing whether possessions will fit into the new property if downsizing, or anticipating that money will have to be spent in adapting the new home can be worrying. Not knowing the new area that you will be living in if you are moving away from your local community can be worrying. Leaving neighbours can be stressful (or a relief!). The thought of having to learn something new – new neighbourhood, where the new shops will be, how to get around the new area – can be daunting. The thought of having new neighbours or new people who you see every day can also be stressful, especially for people who may not previously have had much daily social contact or lived a relatively isolated life. Suddenly having to interact with people every day may be a shock and take some energy, and for people who are not outgoing or sociable, the thought of socialising each day may be exhausting. At the same time, these negatives can be exciting and stimulating for some people, or the reactions can change from one day to the next as the person processes the changes to be made.

There are at least two sides to the move to a new home, looking back and looking forward – the sadness or relief at leaving your old place and old familiar routines, coupled with the anxiety and excitement associated with the process of choosing a new place, and the anxiety of not knowing what the new place will bring.

These emotions can be amplified if the new home is a care home. Not only is the move a change of residence, but the move from individual housing to community living is something that many people do not look forward to. Communal living may be something the person has never experienced before, or only experienced as a child at school or boarding school. The closest to communal living in adulthood may be a hospital episode, which is temporary but also involves group living. The losses are amplified when moving to a care home. The downsizing is substantial if the person has lived in their own home previously. For someone moving from living in their own home with possessions and an environment that they had a large amount of control over, to a care home where their own space shrinks, the emotional aspect of the move can be filled with anxiety, depression and dread. It is common for people to feel a sense of loss and grief over the move, as they have indeed lost a previous environment and lifestyle and may have had to face up to losses associated with health and independence. When these emotions are condensed into a short time period because the decision has to be made quickly, that can make the situation much more challenging as well.

These emotions associated with moving are common and to be expected. Research has shown that autobiographical memories of middle adulthood often centre around any relocations of housing during that period. When people reminisce about what happened to them during the middle years of life, relocation is a common and significant memory (Enz, Pillemer and Johnson 2016). Therefore, it is to be expected that relocation to a care home will become a significant life event and significant memory in the later life of an individual. It is worth trying to make the experience as comfortable as possible and to recognise the achievement of someone who has experienced the move and adapted to their new lifestyle.

Many people fear or dread moving to a care home. One study showed that older people fear moving to a care home more than they fear death (Prince and Butler 2007). In that study,

402 older people were interviewed in the USA. People interviewed said that ageing in place was very important, and over half of the respondents were worried about their ability to remain living independently. Fears that people mentioned were: loss of family, loss of independence, giving up driving and moving into a care home. Isolation, getting sick and death were not as feared. Baby boomers, or children of older people, showed awareness that their parents might feel sad about losing their independence if they had to move from their home. They were also concerned that their parent may dislike living in the home, or be mistreated.

The phenomenon of fear of moving to a care home is so common that in 1992 the North American Nursing Diagnosis Association created a new diagnosis called 'relocation stress syndrome', recognising that the move can be associated with not only psychological but also physiological stress. This syndrome includes symptoms such as anxiety, confusion, hopelessness, depression and loneliness. The symptoms were thought mostly to occur just before, during and up to about three months after relocation (Manion and Rantz 1995).

For many older people, fear of moving to a care home is based on the fear of loss of independence, and loss of control that is assumed to happen when the communal living of an institution is imposed on the individual. Recognising these fears can help older people to start to address them and to work out ways to cope with the feelings.

STRATEGIES TO COPE WITH MOVING

Moving into a care home is a 'stressful life event'. In later life, people can face a number of changes that are challenging. Moving house is one challenge that is considered a stressful life event at any stage of life. It is commonly near the top of the list of stressful life events. The main categories of stressful life events are problems with health, and family problems (Rubio *et al.* 2016). The other most stressful life events people commonly identify are the death of someone close, divorce and major illnesses. Among older people, the types of events that are considered most stressful include death of a family member or friend, illness or injury of a family member or friend, or a non-medical event such as having one's home broken into, or moving house. Many people have recently become bereaved when they move into care, doubling the stressful life events.

Stressful life events can of course occur at any time during adult life. Interestingly, the impact of stressful life events on the risk of developing depression does not change throughout life, so the way stressful life events were coped with earlier in life can be an indication of their likely impact in later life (Kessing, Agerbo and Mortensen 2003). Coping strategies are the ways that people cope with the change that they are experiencing – the methods they use to reduce the stress or the demands of events that they find stressful. Everyone sees the consequences of a stressful life event differently. In one study, for example, people did not consider a heart attack stressful, but retirement was considered stressful (Hardy, Concato and Gill 2002). The consequences of a stressful life event can also vary. Some people find it harder to get everyday things done when stressed, or they stop activities that are usually important to them when they are feeling stressed. These can be symptoms of feeling down or depressed as well as symptoms of stress.

Stressful life events can also have a significant effect on mental health. The stressful event requires the person experiencing the event to adapt to the new situation and it is this process of adaptation that contributes to the stress. Most older people maintain a positive outlook on life and a positive view of themselves as they adapt to stressful life events. This has been referred to as the 'paradox of well-being' – a little like 'looking through rose-tinted glasses'.

> Lord, grant me the serenity to accept the things I cannot change, the courage to change the things I can, and the wisdom to know the difference. (Reinhold Niebuhr, Serenity Prayer, 1986)

Researchers have found that people who are able to use 'flexible goal adjustment' or 'tenacious goal pursuit' seem to weather stressful life events better (Bailly *et al.* 2012). 'Flexible goal adjustment' refers to the ability to adjust to the fact that goals are no longer attainable, and 'tenacious goal pursuit' refers to the ability to deal with attainable goals. These are jargon terms that can be translated: thinking in terms of moving to a care home, it helps to stay positive and keep thinking about the good things about the move. 'Flexible goal adjustment' involves accepting that the goal of staying in previous accommodation is no longer possible or wise, and 'tenacious goal pursuit' involves focusing on things that can be changed about the move rather than things that are outside your control.

Another way of thinking about coping with the move is to consider Niebuhr's Serenity Prayer. The modern psychologists' theories about stressful life events described above seem to have confirmed the merit of Niebuhr's Serenity Prayer. In Niebuhr's terms, 'flexible goal adjustment' means accepting the things you cannot change, i.e. that it is no longer wise or possible to stay in your own home. 'Tenacious goal pursuit' in Niebuhr's terms means having the courage to change the things that you can regarding the move to the care home. This flexibility in thinking about your situation is not something that comes easily to everyone, but it may be a key to moving on and starting to accept and settle in to the change to residential care.

JOSEPHINE'S STORY

Josephine's story illustrates that you should not assume you will be unhappy with the move to a care home. It can work out better than you think. It is very comforting to feel safe and to no longer feel lonely, because people are there to help you.

Josephine migrated from Europe to Australia with her husband and young children several decades ago. She made a new life with her young family, engaging with the local, mostly migrant, community. She is now a proud grandmother and great grandmother. A few years ago, she was widowed and remained in the family home.

Josephine's health, including her mobility, declined gradually. Her family were increasingly concerned that she was living alone. So was Josephine: '...and that's how it started [the process of thinking about moving to care]. I was feeling helpless.' She was also lonely at home, since the loss of her husband, and she felt increasingly vulnerable as her health declined.

After a fall, Josephine was hospitalised, then spent time undergoing rehabilitation. This time away from home prompted Josephine to reconsider her living arrangements. The care residence she moved to was in the same suburb as her family home, and she discovered another resident there was someone she knew from the local community. She has already made a couple of good friends at the residence since moving in. Josephine reflects that making the decision herself to go to a care home probably made it easier to settle in:

'I did it for myself. I did it for my children, because my children all have families... So, I decided to come here. And here, you are never on your own. We have a lot of activities... They give us games, and things to pass the time, you know... I feel OK, I feel I had to do it.'

Josephine acknowledged that it was hard to leave her family home: 'I loved my home, but here, I seem to have forgotten all about it.'

When asked what helped her feel more settled, she replies: 'The nurses, first of all. They're so patient...they are there to give them [residents] help.' Josephine indicates that she can always get help that she needs, and is relieved and happy about this. Josephine also spent time with her family helping to organise the packing up of her family home. She thinks that doing this helped her 'let go' of her home. Her room contains 'homely' touches, including family photographs, her wedding photo and small pieces of favourite furniture.

Josephine feels comfortable and safe in her new place. She states that she is no longer lonely, although she still misses her husband. She describes being able to find someone to have a chat with if she wants to. She also enjoys some time on her own in her room for a few hours each afternoon sitting by the heater, 'It's always warm here,' and she likes looking out of her north-facing window. Josephine says that she feels it is 'pretty good', and describes being free to do what she wants to do.

Maintaining a feeling of control during the decision to move into care has been shown to help with better psychological well-being following the move. People who are excluded from the process of decision making are found to have lower psychological well-being. The feeling of being supported rather than being controlled or directed into decisions is important, even for people whose ability to participate in the decision-making process is not perfect. Forcing an admission into residential care is associated with anger and can increase the mortality rate among people newly admitted to care (Johnson and Bibbo 2014).

Experts suggest that establishing a care plan or an advance care plan can help (see Chapter 3). This can be a difficult conversation or set of conversations to have, and a process that ideally needs to occur over a period of time rather than as a one-off event.

Research shows that it is important to try to maintain as many habits as possible from your previous lifestyle to help to cope with relocation. Reflect on how activities, behaviours, hobbies, routines, relationships, values and attitudes can be continued as much as possible after moving into the care home. For example, if your routine is to have breakfast at 8am each morning, then read the paper, then do some housework, it is worth thinking about how this habit can continue. It may be possible to schedule breakfast and have the paper delivered. Housework may no longer be necessary, but a small part of previous chores such as folding some washing or dusting the bedside table will help to keep things familiar after the move. Maintaining relationships with the same people as much as possible will help. It may no longer be possible to call in to the neighbour down the road, but a phone call or writing a letter at about the same time as was your habit will help to maintain the relationship. This continuity helps to maintain familiarity and to maintain confidence, and to prevent some of the loss of identity associated with moving.

Think about what you can maintain from your life before the care home

- Routines – when and what to eat, shower, sleep, activities you like to do, hobbies.
- Possessions – photos, small furniture, treasures that mean 'home'.
- Clothes – what to wear on certain days, special occasions.
- Social circle – friends and family.

> **Think about things you can let go and no longer need to worry about**
> - Personal care that was becoming difficult.
> - House maintenance, chores, bills.
> - Possessions – large possessions that had become a burden and can be looked after by someone you trust.

FROM THE PERSPECTIVE OF FAMILY AND FRIENDS

Many older people feel pressure from their family and friends to move into a care home. The reasons for such pressure can be numerous. Often well intentioned, family may fear that the person will come to harm if they continue to remain living independently. There may have been one or more incidents where the older person had a mishap, such as a fall that went unattended, or they made a mistake in caring for themselves, such as leaving the gas or the iron on, leading to an accident. Or family may just notice that the older person is starting to have more health issues that are increasingly hard to manage from the family point of view. If they are living far away, there may be the added incentive to relieve family pressure to assist with daily activities. Research has found that caregiver strain is one of the factors that predicts moving into a care home (Heppenstall *et al.* 2014).

Family members may feel torn, seeing both the positives and negatives of moving just like the older person. While their intention may be to keep their relative safe and well cared for, at the same time they may be feeling guilty that they can no longer provide enough care to keep their relative at home, or they may be feeling guilty that they have suggested moving into care when the older person has negative views about care.

Life-changing decisions can bring to the surface lifelong tensions in relationships, and sometimes care home staff can be a target for expressing frustrations associated with these family relationships.

For men caring for their wives, the move of their wife to a care home may mean that two transitions are experienced. The first transition was when they started to adopt the role of carer for their wife. Many older men view their new 'job' of caring differently from that of older women caring for their husbands, for whom their day-to-day role may not have changed significantly from that adopted throughout their life. For the older husband, the caring role he has taken, perhaps running the household for the first time in his life as well as providing personal care, will change again as his wife moves into care. He will lose his role of primary carer again, and have to take on another 'new job' – that of carer who is visiting and monitoring care provided by others. Moving into a care home there may be a transition from intimate care to a new relationship based on friendship (Eriksson and Sandberg 2008). Research suggests that husband primary carers and wife primary carers view their roles very differently.

Next of kin may cope with the transition in a way that is based on previous experiences and relationships with the older person. The relative or family member themselves may feel uncertain about their ability to support their older family member. There may be differences of opinion within the family about who should make decisions, and what the best decision might be, which can make the situation more stressful for all concerned. Family members themselves may be looking to the health care staff for support and guidance in the transition, and staff can have a key role to play in helping the family adjust to their new situations. Family members may continue to feel responsible for their older family member after they have moved into care, and staff will need to help with the family establishing their new roles. One member of the family may have been much more involved in the older person's care than other family members, and the resulting imbalance and communication difficulties will continue to impinge on how the family adjusts to the transition. These family dynamics can be challenging for care home staff to negotiate as well, and they report needing support in learning how to deal with family differences (Doyle and Roberts 2016b).

DISCUSSING MOVING TO A CARE HOME

Most of our conversations with our families and friends cover day-to-day topics, the details of daily life, activities of daily living, news, opinions about events in the local community and around the world. Discussions about what gives meaning to life, emotions experienced in response to events, planning for the future or reviewing the past are a lesser part of most people's conversations, even with people close to them, and the prospect of discussing such significant topics can be daunting. When it comes to discussing personal health, often families and friends are at a loss about how to raise the topic or how to proceed with discussing the topic. As shown here, the topic of residential care can be especially fraught, with social opinions about care invariably negative. How do people raise the topic of moving to a care home?

Points to consider when advising your loved one on moving into a care home
- Get advice from a professional or professional organisation.
- Remember that the cost of care can vary considerably between homes but more expensive is not necessarily better.

- Similar care in the person's home may be available – find out what local services are available.
- Find out what type of care will be most suited for the individual – what are their special needs?
- Look after yourself – caregivers have to consider their own health and it is OK to factor this in to the decision.

Worried family and friends may be met with fierce resistance or anger if the topic of moving to a care home is raised. The older person may be in denial (see Figure 5.1 in Chapter 5), considering that they can take care of themselves despite increasing evidence of a decline in their standard of living or their ability to undertake activities of daily living.

Opening the line of communication early can help to ease the anxiety associated with moving. Discussing what home means, what a care home can provide and what others have done in a similar situation can help both parties to process the issues to be considered. The conversation is not just a one-off event. Having regular conversations will help to discuss the issues from a number of perspectives and allow some time to think about the situation. From the adult child's perspective, phrasing the issue as the child's problem rather than the parent's can open up the parent's thoughts to the impact of their decision on others. If the adult child says, 'I am concerned about... It worries me to see you not being able to manage this...' then the topic may not be viewed as an attempt to remove control from the older person. This is not the time to be directive. By saying 'You have to do this,' or 'You need more help,' the conversation is taking control away from the older person, in which case they are likely to resist.

Over time, the older person may be able to see the situation from other people's points of view and feel less threatened about their independence being removed by a move to care. Most older people do not want to be a burden to their children, and some may not be aware that their adult children are not coping well.

There are no easy strategies to persuade a reluctant older person that moving into care is the probably the best option for everyone. Clearly the older person themselves may feel unsupported if their relative's opinion is different from their own. Asking a parent to 'indulge me' by visiting a care home can start to ease the idea into existence. If a parent is steadfast, the adult child should revisit the topic another time. Sometimes an incident such as a fall can shift an older person's attitudes as they can start to realise that the positives associated with living at home are beginning to be outweighed by the negatives such as safety and quality of life.

If a trusted health care provider or a trusted friend raises the topic of moving into residential care, sometimes the opinion of another person apart from an adult child can help to shift opinions. Discussion with peers or friends of the older person may also help them, although many older people may feel too proud to raise the topic of decreasing independence. If an older person is receiving care services at home, the agency providing the services may give advice about when the higher level of care available in residential care is starting to seem more appropriate. Advice from the agency providing services in the person's home may be more palatable for the older person than advice from their adult child.

Some older people 'try before they buy' by using a respite care visit, which is short term, to see what it feels like to live in residential care for a short time, and the comparison with home living can be enlightening. Having an older person use respite care while an adult child is on holiday so that the holiday is less worrisome can also be an enlightening experience for both parties. A respite care stay that is successful can be the impetus for making the change to permanent residential care. If the older person is willing to visit the home, lengthening the visit to a morning, or an overnight respite visit, can help them to see that the care home is not as bad as they may have imagined.

CHAPTER 3
PLANNING THE MOVE

Planning a move to a care home requires reflecting on your needs and priorities, doing some research and discussing the move with people you trust. If you have not yet spoken with your family doctor (general practitioner, GP), you may be surprised at how much information they can provide about moving to a care home. You may also find that there are options for you to receive subsidised services at home, or you may find that you do not need to move to a care home just yet, but can plan for services at home until you do need to make that move. Increasingly, the government is trying to keep people living in their own homes with the services to assist them to do so. Living at home with community services is not an easy option, especially if living alone, and people sometimes feel relieved to move to communal living after managing alone.

If you know that you need residential care, rather than supported care in your own home, you will most likely be required to have a 'health assessment' by a government-sponsored service, such as a 'care assessment team', or the equivalent. This means a health professional or team of health professionals will provide an assessment to determine your current and anticipated future health and social care needs.

The assessment is usually free, and the process helps ensure that a suitable level of care with appropriate services can be identified for you. Your family doctor will be able to tell you how to arrange this assessment, and some governments require that your family doctor initiate this assessment.

A decision pathway for moving into residential care

- Think about what extra support you need to make life more comfortable.
- Obtain a care needs assessment.
- Decide on what is most important to you, and ask if the care home can accommodate that.
- Consider the financial costs – get advice from a reputable residential care financial adviser.
- Organise your affairs – have a current will, consider advance care planning, explore appointing a substitute decision maker and financial power of attorney.
- Make a shortlist of possible suitable care homes.
- Check inspection reports, ask friends and family for their recommendations.
- Visit some care homes that may be suitable for you and ask about providing the things that are most important to you.

HOW DO YOU KNOW WHICH CARE HOME WILL SUIT YOU?

Phoning, emailing or writing to homes that might be suitable in your local area to ask for specific information, or looking up their websites on the internet is a good place to start. Ask about the level of care provided, the fees and any waiting lists. Keep a file of your research. If you have the opportunity to choose a home, the choice can be hard as there seem to be so many factors to take into account. There are many checklists available to help you to assess each care home that you visit (internet sources of checklists and websites with other useful information are listed at the back of this book). Some checklists are very detailed, and some are specialised, such as those for someone living with dementia. Using one of these checklist guides can help when comparing homes, but the guides are general and will not take into account your own priorities – no care home will be perfect and tick all the boxes, and not every home will suit everyone. It is important to think about what matters most to you before choosing a care home: just as when moving to a new house, no home is likely to have everything you want, so some compromises on less important aspects of the home may have to be made.

Common themes in checklists for judging the suitability of care homes are shown in the following text box.

When comparing care homes, some aspects that you can check are:
- location and accessibility for friends and family
- first impressions, surroundings
- staffing levels or training
- whether day-to-day care provision will provide what you need
- social life and activities available
- food and catering
- contracts and fees
- provisions for couples and privacy
- environment, atmosphere
- medical and special supports
- provisions for visitors, and sitting areas to entertain them.

Visiting a care home can be confronting and depressing. We do not feel old inside, and some older people report feeling shocked when they see the wrinkles and grey hair on the person in the mirror! Being confronted with a lounge room full of old people who seem to be lacking in vitality, purpose or engagement can seem depressing. Is that my future, what I am going to be like, or my family member? When making visits to potential residences it can help to recognise that this is a significant life event that is being experienced, and that the visit may raise upsetting emotions. Be kind to yourself in this visiting phase. Taking some specific questions, a checklist or a notepad to write down observations will help to give some structure to the visit. Look at the individuals in the home rather than seeing a group of people who are all the same. Say hello to those you meet, when appropriate, and perhaps have a short chat about their home. Some homes have a friendlier, more relaxed atmosphere than others, and this 'first impressions' feeling is worth noting. Meeting the care manager or some senior staff is important in helping to work out what the home will be like. If you warm to the senior staff then that is an indication that the home may be a good one for you. Choosing a home in the same area you have lived in will help it to feel familiar, but sometimes it is not possible to stay in the same location or the local home is not suitable.

The quality of homes varies considerably. A good quality home will allow for person-centred care (see Chapter 7), so that you can maintain interests and your own routines to some extent. Your rights should be respected, including the right to make choices. There should be some opportunity to maintain your interests, and the right to choose in many aspects of daily life. The physical environment of the home should be homely rather than hotel or hospital like. There is a myriad of information to take in, but bear in mind what your own priorities are and ask about those. For example, you may be able to adjust to having a shower in the morning instead of the evening, but would definitely prefer to have breakfast in your room each day. If this is an important detail for you, note it down and ask about that detail. No care home is likely to have everything you would like so it is worth reflecting on what is most important to you, what you can live with and what you can compromise on, what you would not be able to tolerate and what would make life better.

WHO ELSE CAN HELP ME?

After speaking with your family doctor or health professional, there are other sources of information to help with the move to a care home, including:

- Checklists to help with viewing care home facilities (see a sample at the end of this book).
- Internet websites that discuss factors to consider (but be aware that not all the websites have reliable information – choose well-known organisations); there are some listed in Appendix 1 of this book.
- Local council or city offices – your local city, state and national government agencies may also have a telephone helpline and website for older people and their families, including those contemplating residential care services. Your local city or government offices will also be able to provide you with telephone numbers and websites of relevant care agencies in your area.
- Care providers – in addition, care providers usually have their own websites to browse. They provide a contact telephone number and invite you to visit their care homes. Many care homes are part of a large organisation supporting several homes, and you can contact them by telephone to ask any questions, either general or specific,

about moving to residential care. The internet is a good source of information, but it may provide you with too much irrelevant information, like searching for a needle in a haystack.

Managers of care homes can also provide information to you over the telephone or when you visit, and there is no obligation for you to make a quick decision about moving in. In fact, care homes are constantly getting enquiries from the community and they usually have well-developed resources and services for providing information.

In some areas, you can directly contact care assessment teams, or their equivalent; the people who carry out the assessments of older people regarding their suitability for residential care can also provide helpful and impartial information to assist you with what you need to do, and in what order.

For families of older people considering residential care, it may be helpful to speak with a calm and trusted friend who has been through the process recently with their own relative. However, the more people you ask, the more confusing the process of getting information about residential care can become. It is helpful to think about the older person's own main priorities during this process and follow the course that best suits their priorities rather than yours, if you are a family member or friend – the two may not always be the same.

At this time, it is important to take care of yourself. Listening to well-meaning others recount their unhappy experiences about care homes may not be the most supportive thing for you right now (or ever!), but constructive and informative advice based on personal experience from someone reassuring, whom you trust, can be very helpful.

Summary points for planning your move

- Talk with your family about moving to a care home, in a gentle, unhurried way.
- Ask a trusted health professional or your family doctor about what you need to do and where to get relevant information from regarding financing residential care.
- Reflect on what your own priorities are, what you could compromise on and what you would definitely like to experience.
- Explore the cost of residential care and determine the best way for you to afford the care you need.
- Contact the residential care section of your local council (municipality) in person or by telephone and discuss your care needs and concerns.
- Telephone your local government residential care sections, and read their websites on care homes.
- Ask a knowledgeable friend or relative to help you, or your local community health centre or neighbourhood house centre if you have one. This information can be difficult to understand without someone to help explain it all to you. Social workers at your hospital or community health centre may be able to help.
- Choose carefully whom you seek out to discuss their care home experiences as often people will only recount negative experiences.
- Remember, you are not alone, and that it is OK to get as much help and support as you need.

FINANCIAL AND LEGAL ISSUES

Part of the move to residential care will involve finding out as early as possible what financial assistance is available to you, so you can live as comfortably as possible. In many western countries, including the UK, Australia, New Zealand, Canada and the USA, the government subsidises the costs of older people receiving residential care, although the amount of subsidy varies. General information is available from government websites and agencies (see Appendix 1 at the end of this book), and then you will have specific questions for individual care homes that you approach.

You may receive a subsidy from the government in addition to what you can afford to pay through your income and assets, or the government may pay much of the cost of your care if you have limited income and assets.

Questions to ask about finance and residential care
Fees and contracts vary a great deal, and many are challenging to understand. Ask to see a copy of the home's contract and terms and conditions, and have someone you trust review them, then discuss anything that is not clear. A lawyer or community legal centre, or an experienced social worker may also be able to help answer your questions, or help you clarify further questions for the care home. If you are using a checklist for choosing a care home in your local region/area, it will have some specific questions about fees and contracts. There are some general questions to consider:
- What fees are involved?
- How frequently are fees reviewed?

- What is included in the weekly charge and what will need to be paid for separately?
- Are valuables covered by the home's insurance?
- Are fees reviewed or altered? How often?

Learning about the financial aspects of moving to a care home can be confusing, even for people who normally manage many complexities in their lives. As well as thinking about the financial side, there are some important legal aspects to consider. Arguably, one of the most important aspects is whom you can trust to make decisions about your health and medical care in the event that you become too ill to make such decisions, either temporarily or permanently.

Here, we wish to raise important related issues regarding decision making, appointing financial powers of attorney and generally allowing others to help you with your financial and business affairs, and with your health and social care.

DECISION MAKING ABOUT YOUR FUTURE CARE

We usually expect to continue to make our own decisions about our care as we get older, but sometimes this is not possible, due to health reasons. Many people live in the hope that they will continue to be independent, including in their medical treatment and health care decision making. Increasingly, many people moving to a care home have illnesses, such as dementia, that may eventually or do already affect their ability to think clearly. This means that they or their family can anticipate a time when it is important that the people caring for them or their family members know what sort of care they would or would not want, based on the affected person's values and beliefs.

Person-centred care, which means care that focuses in a 'tailored' way on the needs of the person moving into care, based on their values and beliefs (Dow *et al.* 2006), can be more likely to happen if a person has an 'advance care plan'. More and more, care homes encourage residents to participate in 'advance care planning' if they are legally competent to do so and do not already have an advance care plan. Many governments now insist that care homes ask people if they have an advance care plan, and assist people who do not have one to develop one that reflects the values and beliefs about the care they would or would not want.

ADVANCE CARE PLANNING

Advance care planning is an umbrella term that can include making an 'advance care directive'. It involves thinking about, discussing and writing down what care arrangements you prefer, and ideally the values and beliefs that influence them, in anticipation of a time when you may be unable to express your future health care or medical treatment wishes. It should be an ongoing discussion process, rather than a one-off conversation (McGlade *et al.* 2017; Thomas and Lobo 2011).

Advance care planning involves more than just you and your family doctor or nurse 'having a talk'. If done properly in a health care or care home setting, advance care planning requires visiting health professionals or staff to have special training and communication skills. Family members and very close friends may also need to be involved in your conversations about future care wishes, and any decisions about future care need to be shared, at least verbally, among the important people in your life, so that everyone is clear and 'on the same page' about your wishes if a critical health situation arises for you. Specially trained health professionals helping with advance care planning can also ensure that the significant people in your life are included in the process or, at least, informed of the your wishes, if you wish them to be.

Advance care planning can be done in a number of ways. Importantly, any advance care plan, either simple or more detailed, is only good *if it is legally valid, likely to be followed, and if it most truly reflects the current wishes for the current circumstances of the person.* This is why advance care plans tend to work best when they are fairly simple and flexible, the existence of the plan is known by all concerned, and is easily accessible. It is also best if the plan is reviewed periodically, and the person with the advance care plan remains in the care of those who are clear about what the care plan is, such as the staff and visiting health professionals at a care home. Unfortunately, there is limited evidence so far of the effectiveness of advance care plans to increase the likelihood of patient preferences for future care being followed, especially for people living with cognitive impairment (Robinson *et al.* 2012). If a person is moved to somewhere else for care, and the staff at the new location are not familiar with the person or with their care plan, there is a higher likelihood that their wishes may not be known or followed, and they may receive unwanted care. This sometimes happens, for example, when a person is sent to hospital from a care home.

LEONARD'S STORY

Leonard's story illustrates that it is important to plan for people who you know and trust to assist you if a situation arises where you are unable to make decisions for yourself.

Leonard was 77, lived alone with little family support and eventually decided, with the help and agreement of his family doctor, that he would need to move to a care home as it was becoming impossible for him to manage at home and he was feeling quite unsafe living alone since his Parkinson's disease had got worse. Leonard was concerned that the staff at his care home would not know him, and he did not want to lose control of decision making about his treatment completely. His family doctor informed him after chatting about who would be his 'default' legal substitute decision maker, that Leonard should find out from the Office of the Public Advocate (in Australia). Leonard contacted the Office and was informed that his nephew, Ian, would in fact be contacted and invited to make decisions about his medical care, as his 'person responsible' if Leonard became unable to do so. Leonard was surprised to learn this, although he had never really thought about who would advocate for him, if he could not make treatment decisions. He had not seen his nephew for two years, even though he was his closest blood relative. They only talked on the telephone every few months.

Leonard realised that his nephew, Ian, would know very little about what Leonard would want or not want regarding treatment if Ian had to make a decision about his care. Leonard assumed that his family doctor would make any such decisions for him. Leonard approached his family doctor and local priest about who might be his substitute decision maker (SDM), as he decided he needed to appoint someone whom he trusted to make decisions that would accord with his values and beliefs. His kind family doctor agreed that he was happy to be appointed as SDM, and his local priest, Father Ray, who also knew his doctor, indicated that he was also happy to support Leonard, and the doctor, should the need arise. Leonard made a point of meeting both his doctor and his priest separately and together to discuss what treatment he would and wouldn't want in future. With the assistance of the local solicitor, Leonard appointed his doctor as his SDM and the paperwork for this was also given to Father Ray, the care home he moved to and to his nephew, Ian. Leonard felt much more comfortable after this advance care planning process had taken place and the care home staff were informed of his plan, and had copies of his documentation.

He continues to chat regularly with Father Ray and his doctor since his move. The staff at his care home are also getting to know him better as he has become happier since the move.

ADVANCE CARE DIRECTIVES

An advance care plan can be more detailed, and may include making an 'advance (care) directive' about your future care. An 'advance care directive' means a specific direction or instruction made in advance that has a basis in law, and the law will vary depending on the area in which you live.

An advance care directive can include instructions about what sort of care you do or do not want, in what circumstances, and who you would wish to make medical treatment decisions on your behalf. In Victoria, Australia, a new law, the Medical Treatment Planning and Decisions Act 2016, will enable Victorians to appoint a medical decision maker and also to make an advance directive, known as an 'instructional directive'. For more information about this particular law, and to see examples of advance care directives, see Compassion in Dying (UK) and Office of the Public Advocate (Australia) in Appendix 1. If you are interested in advance care directives (also known as 'advance decisions or living wills'), you need to ask for advice from a lawyer, your community legal centre, community health centre, a social worker, your family doctor or another trusted and knowledgeable person, to find out more about this type of advance directive (Lobo and Thomas 2011). The following is an example of a legal document from the Medical Treatment Act 1988 (VIC) that has been used in Victoria, Australia, to enable people to make an advance care directive to refuse certain medical treatment related to a current medical condition.

Medical Treatment Act 1988
SCHEDULE 1
Sections 3, 5(2)
Refusal of Treatment Certificate: Competent Person

We certify that we are satisfied:
(a) that . . . . [name of patient] has clearly expressed or indicated a decision, in relation to a current condition, to refuse –
*medical treatment generally;
or
*medical treatment, being . . . .'. . . . .
[specify particular kind of medical treatment];

(b) that the patient's decision is made voluntarily and without inducement or compulsion;

(c) that the patient has been informed about the nature of his/her current condition to an extent which is reasonably sufficient to enable him/her to make a decision about whether or not to refuse medical treatment generally or of a particular kind (as the case requires) and that he/she has appeared to understand that information;

(d) that the patient is of sound mind and has attained the age of 18 years.
Dated: . . . .
Signed: . . . . [Registered medical practitioner]
Signed: . . . . [Another person]

Patient's current condition
The patient's current condition is . . . .
. . . . [describe condition]
Dated: . . . .
Signed: . . . .
[To be signed by the same registered medical practitioner]

Source: Office of the Public Advocate www.publicadvocate.vic.gov.au
(permission granted)

Figure 3.1: Example of an advance care directive

Another type of advance care directive is the formal appointment of someone as 'substitute decision maker'. This role may also be called an enduring medical power of attorney, durable power of attorney, or proxy decision maker, depending on the law where you live (Lobo and Thomas *et al.* 2011). In England and Wales, an appointed substitute decision maker is known as a Lasting Power of Attorney for Health and Welfare (LPA). Currently, the law concerning health treatment decision making where you live will identify who the 'person responsible' is, who would be legally responsible for making treatment decisions for you. This is the legal 'default system' for identifying who would speak for you and make decisions for you when you cannot, and such systems exist in all western countries. Do you know who the law recognises as your 'person responsible' (or equivalent)?

Currently, most older people do not participate in advance care planning in the general community (Gould *et al.* 2015), but for people living in care homes, advance care planning is recognised as relevant and helpful (Mignani *et al.* 2017). In most cases, the default decision-making system works well, but sometimes, a family member you do not know well, or do not like, may legally be the person asked to make decisions for you, or there may be conflicting views among your family members as to what treatment you would want in particular circumstances. If you are in this situation or you do not have close family, appointing a 'substitute decision maker' might be a good option for you. The appointment may give you peace of mind that someone who knows you and with whom you have discussed your values and beliefs regarding your future health care decisions would be involved in decision making concerning you. This can also be relevant for people in gay or lesbian relationships, where their family of origin refuses to accept the relationship or recognise the same-sex partner as 'legitimately' their partner.

Figure 3.2 is an example of a legal document from the Medical Treatment Act 1988 (VIC) that has been used in Victoria,

Australia, to appoint an 'enduring medical power of attorney' (substitute decision maker), who can make medical treatment decisions for the person who is no longer able to make their own such decisions (note that this document is due to be updated in the near future; check the website www.publicateadvocate.vic. gov.au).

ENDURING POWER OF ATTORNEY (MEDICAL TREATMENT)
THIS ENDURING POWER OF ATTORNEY is given on the
day of . . . . [Print date, month and year here]
by . . . .[Print your full name here]
of . . . .[Print your address here]
under Section 5A of the Medical Treatment Act 1988.

Cross out the following option if you also wish to appoint an alternate agent.
1. I APPOINT
. . . .[Print the full name of your agent here]
of . . . .[Print your agent's address here] to be
my agent.

OR, Cross out the following option if you do not wish to appoint an alternate agent.
1. I APPOINT
. . . .[Print the full name of your agent here]
of . . . .[Print your agent's address here] to be
my agent.
and . . . .[Print the full name of your alternative agent here]
of . . . .[Print your alternative agent's address here] to be
my alternative agent.

2. I AUTHORISE my agent or, if applicable, my alternative agent, to make decisions about medical treatment on my behalf.

3. I REVOKE all other enduring powers of attorney (medical treatment) previously given by me.
SIGNED, SEALED AND DELIVERED by: . . . .
[Sign your name here]

We . . . . [Print your witnesses' names here] each
believe that . . . . [Print your name here] in making
this enduring power of attorney (medical treatment) is of sound mind and
understands the import of this document.

WITNESSED by:

. . . . [Witnesses sign here]

Person authorised to witness statutory declarations

. . . . [print your witness' name here]

. . . . [Address of witness]

Other witness

. . . . [print your witness' name here]

. . . . [Address of witness]

Source: Office of the Public Advocate www.publicadvocate.vic.gov.au
(permission granted)

Figure 3.2: Example of a form to appoint an 'enduring medical power of attorney'

COPYRIGHT © State of Victoria, Australia Copyright in all legislation of the Parliament of the State of Victoria, Australia, is owned by the Crown in right of the State of Victoria, Australia. DISCLAIMER This product or service contains an unofficial version of the legislation of the Parliament of State of Victoria. The State of Victoria accepts no responsibility for the accuracy and completeness of any legislation contained in this product or provided through this service.

WHO MAKES AN ADVANCE CARE PLAN?

People without cognitive impairment are legally able to make an advance care plan, including advance care directives, such as the appointment of a substitute decision maker or refusal of treatment (McGlade *et al.* 2017). People can and do change their mind as their lives progress, and circumstances can arise that are not anticipated, so any written decisions about future care may need to be revisited regularly, and certainly after any significant change in the health of the person living in the care home (Neher 2004). Your family doctor or a health professional such as a neuropsychologist is best placed to make a professional assessment *if there is any doubt* about your cognitive capacity.

For people moving to residential care who have a cognitive impairment and who do not have an advance care plan, it is important for their family members to nevertheless try and include the person with cognitive impairment in a conversation about what is important to them and what treatment they would or would not want (McGlade *et al.* 2017). This should be done in a way that does not cause the person distress, and only if it is culturally appropriate to do so (Ke *et al.* 2017). Some people with cognitive impairment may, however, not be capable of involvement in such a conversation due to the deterioration in their cognitive health. If a person can be included in such discussions about their care, it can help to ensure that the person feels they have knowledge and some sense of control over the decision-making process. If someone has memory loss, some important outcomes of decisions may need to be written down for that person, so they can be reminded and reassured when necessary.

HOW DO I GO ABOUT MAKING AN ADVANCE CARE PLAN?

The proportion of people with advance care planning living in residential care has increased rapidly in many western countries due to the expectations of government and care organisations. In some areas, having an advance care plan is tied to care home accreditation (required quality standards), and advance care planning is deemed by government as a sign of 'good' care being provided at a care home.

Some people may choose to write something like the following letter, which is valid in common law. In practice, however, care staff are usually more inclined to follow an authoritative formal 'form', rather than a handwritten letter due to their lack of understanding of the common law. The education of many care staff has some way to go in this area. It is not uncommon for even senior care staff and some medical practitioners to lack an understanding of the possible validity of handwritten documents provided by patients and residents. Things are improving in this regard, but more slowly than is required by growing demand.

If you wish to handwrite a letter about your future treatment decisions, seek legal advice before doing so, to ensure your letter has the best chance of being as clear and unambiguous as possible, and so that your country's prevailing laws are taken into consideration. An example of a simple letter indicating your preferred medical treatment decision maker is as follows:

Dear (Friend or family member's name)

Thank you for spending the time listening to me today, and for discussing what sort of health care and medical treatment decisions I would want, based on my personal beliefs and values.

As you are my trusted friend, I now feel very confident that you also understand what is important to me, and I feel confident that I can trust you to make the right medical and treatment decision for me, if the need arises for you to do so. I have taken the necessary legal steps to appoint you as my legal medical treatment decision maker, too, should I become unable, temporarily or permanently, to make my own such decisions.

MOVING INTO RESIDENTIAL CARE

I thank you for your love and ongoing care of me.

Yours sincerely

[Your name, date of birth and the date of the letter being written/conversation taking place, preferably in your own legible handwriting]

Speaking to the person you legally appoint as your 'substitute decision maker', as well as your other close family and carers, is a simple and effective way of advance care planning, if communication is open, honest and regular. Writing a letter similar to the example above may provide extra comfort to a person when considering who would make decisions for them if they could not. The provision of comfort and a sense of control is part of what advance care planning can best offer, and this should be remembered by care home staff who are welcoming a new resident.

Care homes keep copies of advance care plans, which may include advance care directives, in their files or in a prominent place so they are easily accessible for staff.

Writing a very long, detailed or vague advance care plan that cannot be applied to all circumstances arising in the future is problematic for your decision makers (family, any substitute decision maker and your health care team). It may also lack legal validity. It is hard to anticipate every likely scenario in the future. For some people, a complex advance care plan including an advance directive or advance directives might be best, but for the majority this is likely not to be the case. A suitably experienced lawyer, your family doctor or your medical specialist might best be able to advise you about whether an advance care directive or appointing a substitute decision maker and having a 'refusal of treatment' certificate (or your country, province or state's equivalent) is likely to increase your chances of getting treatment that best accords with your values and beliefs and avoids you being subjected to care you would not want.

The preferred style of decision making for some people is based less on 'individual' decision making, and more on 'collective' or group decision making between trusted family members, or a designated family member (Ke *et al.* 2017). This might apply to your family situation, and this is why care home staff and family decision makers need to know what the person moving to care might value in their future treatment, and what they may not value, so that the right decision can be made for the person.

Very well-meaning family members can make decisions based on what they honestly think is in the 'best interests' of the person living in residential care, but sometimes they can be mistaken, due to the stress and emotional complexity of coping with their loved one living in a care home. Instead, they might make decisions based on what *they* want, rather than what their family member would choose in the circumstances. It should also be remembered that even substitute decision making, where a person is legally able to make substitute decisions based on what they think the person would choose for themselves in the circumstances if they were able to, can choose care contrary to what the person would have preferred (Shalowitz, Garrett-Mayer and Wendler 2006).

Initiating discussions and talking about anticipated serious illness, death and funeral arrangements can be considered very rude, disrespectful, inappropriate, taboo or likely to bring bad luck (Ke *et al.* 2017). It is therefore important to let the care home know how you or your relative would like to have decisions about their health and medical care made. Who would normally make such decisions, and how would such decisions normally be made? For example, would it be a round-table discussion among several family members, or just a few, or just one?

Many health professionals and consumer advocacy groups argue strongly that having an advance care plan can be a comfort for people living with ill health and increasingly fragile health, giving them peace of mind that they will get the treatment that fits with their culture, beliefs and life values. But, every family is different, and so are its individual members. It is important that all care staff know what you or your family member would want, and how such decisions should be made if the person moving to a care home can no longer decide for themselves.

For families that *can* have discussions about future care, it can be a very helpful way of learning more about the values and beliefs that a person would want respected if others were making decisions for them, and advance care planning can be a helpful tool.

ELDER ABUSE

As we get older, circumstances can force us to rely more on others than we have in the past. For most people, there are trusted family and friends who are available and only too willing to help us out in a genuinely loving and caring way. If you are in a position where the people who are helping you out are not necessarily the most trustworthy or caring, you can become vulnerable to what is termed 'elder abuse'. Of course, some people think the people who are helping them are trustworthy, and some learn the hard way that this is in fact not the case. Elder abuse might be subtle, or it can be more obvious. If you suspect you may be experiencing elder abuse, trust your feelings and get confidential help.

If you are worried about the care you are receiving, or if you wish to learn more about protecting yourself and your assets, seek advice from a trusted professional, such as your family doctor or a social worker at your local hospital or community centre or a national support telephone helpline (see Appendix 1 at the back of this book). There are some links at the back of the book about what elder abuse is, how to avoid it and what can be done about it. It should be stressed that, while it is not a common phenomenon, sadly it is not rare.

SUMMARY POINTS ABOUT ADVANCE CARE PLANNING

- An advance care plan is designed to help you make decisions for future care, at a time when you may not be able to speak for yourself regarding your treatment wishes due to illness.
- If you or your family member are used to making important decisions as a group, or, traditionally expect that a person in your family is the family 'decision maker', it may be necessary to legally appoint that person as your substitute decision maker to ensure that they would speak for you if you were unable to make decisions for yourself. This appointment can usually be done either for free, or inexpensively, by filling in a proforma or writing a letter with the assistance of a community legal centre, a senior rights advocacy service, a community social worker or a lawyer.
- It is also important to let the care home you are moving to know how you and your family wish future treatment decisions to be made.
- You are not obliged to participate in a formal advance care planning process if you do not wish to. You should, however, ask questions about who, in law, would be your 'default' substitute decision maker if you were unable to make your own health and social care decisions.
- A lawyer, community legal service, your family doctor or a government residential care advice line may assist you with finding more information (see Appendix 1 at the end of this book).

- It is important to discuss with your 'default' or appointed substitute decision maker, and significant others, what your values and beliefs are that would influence your future treatment wishes from time to time. You may also consider writing a letter, making a recording or completing another form of advance care directive.
- If advance care planning is important to you, ask the care home you decide to move to about their advance care planning policy and what processes and systems are in place to help ensure that your advance care planning is reviewed regularly.

MOVING TO A CARE HOME UNEXPECTEDLY

Even with the best planning, the move into residential care can happen unexpectedly, precipitated by a health crisis or a sudden change in circumstances. In Switzerland, one study found that 43 per cent of older people are admitted to care homes after hospital discharge (Koppitz *et al.* 2017). The estimated percentages vary from one country to the next. In the USA, the percentage is lower at 32.5 per cent and in Germany only 19 per cent (Koppitz *et al.* 2017). For people who have to move unexpectedly, the decision to move into residential care is often hard for the person concerned to process. There can be a sense of urgency as pressure to leave hospital and vacate the expensive hospital bed pushes decisions to be made quickly, and not in a 'person-centred' way. In those circumstances, the older person themselves can sometimes only be included passively in decisions, with those around them making decisions for them while they are feeling unwell.

For someone without a close relative or someone who can advocate for them, the situation can be especially difficult, as the older person is swept along by other people's priorities and decision making. Many people in these circumstances find that relocation to a care home seems involuntary and out of their control. The unplanned nature of the decision can be especially difficult to absorb. Being unwell because of an acute health event makes the situation even more challenging as it can be hard to think clearly. However, everyone has the right to decide as many aspects of the move as they are able to for themselves. Older people who are cognitively unimpaired cannot be moved into a care home against their will, but when in hospital, feeling unwell, without their home and possessions around them, they can find the decision to move very challenging to approach in a calm, rational way. The older person in these circumstances is usually quite vulnerable and needs extra support to navigate such a major life change. Staff and family who acknowledge the difficult circumstances and the challenge of making decisions while feeling unwell can help the older person to feel supported. The person needs someone to advocate on their behalf, and it is useful to think about who this person might be well in advance of any health event, and to discuss the situation with them as well.

Some relevant questions
- Who will ensure I maintain my dignity and have my human rights respected if I become unwell while living in a care home?
- What can I do now to let others know what health and medical care I do and do not want?
- Can my family spend my money/sell my house/ property without me knowing if I move to a care home?
- Can I still make legal decisions about finances and health care if I have mild dementia?
- Who can legally make which type of decisions for me, if I am unable to?
- What is a 'financial power of attorney', and what decisions can they make?

- What is 'elder abuse' in relation to finances and my human rights?
- What if I run out of money while living in care?
- Who is helping me with my banking and money management? Will this change if I move to a care home?
- Will I be given treatment I do not want, or sent to hospital if I don't wish this to happen?

If an older person experiences a series of hospital admissions, that can be a predictor of admission into residential care as it is often a sign that the person's health has deteriorated. However, it is only one predictor, and there are other factors that are involved as well.

Moving into a care home from hospital
- Ask for information from the hospital – staff may have a leaflet or guide for patients, families or carers.
- Use a checklist of what each home provides to help you prioritise your needs and decide which of the homes on offer will suit you best (see Appendix 1 for some checklists to help you to think about what your priorities are).
- Bear in mind that you might need to move to a temporary location until a vacancy becomes available in your preferred home. Research has shown that it is better for your health to avoid long stays in hospital so it is best to wait for your care home place outside the hospital environment.

When the move is unexpected, choices may be limited by the timing and by lack of information about alternatives. In these circumstances, learning about what to expect at the care home before arriving there can help. The day of the move can be especially difficult. Showing the older person photos of where they are going, involving them in the process of moving away from the hospital and acknowledging the role of the nursing and medical staff can give the older person a sense of control. Having the new room furnished with some familiar belongings may help with feelings of lost identity but, if possible, the choice of these belongings should be made in consultation with the older person so that they can feel in control. For example, a favourite piece of furniture and a bedspread or comforter may make the room seem more like the resident's 'home', and decorating the room with some familiar objects, favourite colours and textures – anything that will help the person feel more comfortable with their new surroundings – can provide comfort, but this needs to be approached sensitively as the older person may feel that their personal things have been taken over by the person doing the decorating. Giving the new resident choice in where to put things may help. This is also important for residents with a cognitive impairment, including dementia.

If the older person is able to go home to 'say goodbye' to their home, some people will find this process helpful in their grieving process but the event may be painful and requires careful handling, again in consultation with the older person. Pastoral carers from the care home may be able to assist with this process and be with the older person as this 'goodbye' becomes part of the 'ceremonies' that mark the transition. Some older people may be ready to help sort their possessions, or to help in organising disposal of possessions such as furniture that will no longer need to be used. The timing of this process needs to be considered carefully, as the process of adjustment may take some time.

If someone is coming straight from hospital, then a period of time to recover is required before the added stress of saying goodbye to possessions is tackled. This ordering of steps can help the older person to feel as though they are leading the process of moving, but it will not be the approach that suits everyone, and may be of limited value where a person has short-term memory loss. Communicating with the older person and involving them in decisions as much as possible will assist the person to feel more in control even though the decision about returning home may have been presented to them as a 'fait accompli'.

What is most important is that the resident still has some sort of connection to their 'previous' life, including their home and community, through what ever means works best for them, whether this is possessions, contact with neighbours, news about events or maintaining a role that is similar to their previous life, however small. People may need the opportunity to develop a sense of 'resolution' about that life chapter and the start of their next chapter. This can take extra time and care when the resident feels they were unprepared for a move they had little choice about. This may include a person who has a cognitive impairment and, due to memory loss, can no longer recall the move or their involvement in it.

Some people who have been part of a religious community find continuing with that spiritual support is helpful. From a spiritual perspective, offering the person prayer or other religious activities if that has been part of their life previously can help them to adjust, especially if they have not been well. For everyone, regardless of whether they have been spiritually aware in the past, it is important to be 'present' for the new resident, visit them frequently and listen to them as much as they need, and to acknowledge their experience. This conveys to residents that they are cared for and respected.

Sometimes, surprisingly, the quick decision of an unexpected move can be easier to accept. If someone was socially isolated at their own home, then moving into care where there are people around can improve feelings of safety. If the decision to move is precipitated by a health crisis, it can be easier to accept when a sudden deterioration makes it impossible to continue to live independently, whereas a slow gradual decline in living independently can make it harder to let go. Some older people accept the authority of their medical doctor as knowing what is best for them, and can feel cared for if the decision is taken out of their hands. In circumstances where the decision is sudden, communication with others is still important, and the older person needs to be involved in the decision rather than feeling as though it was their family, doctor or health professional who decided for them. Taking control of the decision away leaves the person at risk of becoming depressed about their loss of identity and control. The individual has the right to feel as though they made an informed decision to move to care, even when they are taking advice from a trusted medical professional.

MALCOLM'S STORY

Malcolm's story illustrates that it is important to ask for help and let those close to you know how you are feeling. In the care home, some people are trained to understand and support people in their transition to residential care. They can help you to work out strategies to help you to feel safer and provide practical assistance at a difficult time of change.

Malcolm had been contemplating eventual admission to a care home due to a gradual decline in his health and his mobility. However, Malcolm's move occurred several months earlier than he expected.

His health got worse, forcing him into hospital. For various reasons, Malcolm moved suddenly to the care home directly from hospital, with, he felt, no practical or emotional preparation, and before he was able to speak with his family. He recalls feeling 'totally isolated [and]...in supreme stress', due to the quick move to residential care and, after five months, he is only just starting to feel as if things are settling down into a routine.

Malcolm recalls moving into an unfamiliar and almost empty room. He states, 'As far as treatment was concerned, there was no harshness about it...I can't do anything but praise everyone here, and, er, particularly...Tess (the pastoral care practitioner), I think it might have been fate; she has been so good... She checks up on me pretty frequently.'

Soon after the move he became ill again, requiring more hospitalisation. This further compounded his bewilderment at the sudden, significant changes in his life. Malcolm can now joke about moving into resdiential care, and being reminded of the passing years. 'I have noticed some older people here,' he says, grinning. 'The thing is, I've walked into the bathroom and looked in the mirror and thought, "Who's that old bloke?"'

Malcolm has loving but limited family support, and has found it difficult to adjust to life in a care home while at the same time organising his financial affairs. He believes it is more difficult to adjust as you get older, but he did notice that when in hospital after moving to the care home, he told the hospital staff on discharge that he was 'going home'. He thought this was a good sign. Over the last five months, he has had his family visit and bring him in some things from his previous home, which he helped to pack up and clear of its contents. He says this helped him say goodbye to his house.

Malcolm's room is no longer bare. He has several photographs of family members, including his children and grandchildren, placed around the room. He looks out on a spacious and sunny courtyard that has brilliant coloured flowers. He does not know many of his 'neighbours' at the residence yet, as he has not engaged with them very much while coming to terms with all the change that has happened. He has, however, kept in contact with family and friends, sometimes using the telephone. He maintains his interests, too, explaining, 'I like study, and, um, I've more or less studied into my 60s and I'm always watching documentaries and those types of things to keep up to date... A friend [and I], we've developed an interest in quantum physics, as you do [laughs]; Stephen Hawking, that type of thing.'

Malcolm reflects that he has had a lot of support from the staff. He remembers that the social worker from the hospital was also very supportive; he explained to Malcolm what to expect on his admission to the care home, and how the process of admission works. Malcolm has now discovered that someone he knows well and trusts has a relative living at the home and this gives him more comfort and reassurance that he is in the right place.

CHAPTER 4

SETTLING IN AND GETTING THE SUPPORT YOU NEED

Everyone is different and the journey and transition to residential care is unique for each new resident and their family.

PASTORAL CARE PRACTITIONER

Once the move into a care home has been made, expect that there will be a period of time of settling in and working out how best to live life in new surroundings. The move to a care home may bring with it a range of emotions, including grief, that can make the person moving to care feel unsettled, uncertain and even fearful about their future. It can also be a confusing time for new residents learning about the new daily routines, especially so if they have a cognitive impairment. If the move to residential care has been decided on and acted on very quickly, new residents and their families have little time to adjust emotionally to the move. Additionally, some members of a family may have differing views about the necessity of residential care for their relative, and where families do have differing views, the transition for the resident can be more challenging. Staff are aware of these special issues for new residents and their families, and can help by providing extra support both during the transition and the ongoing period.

Everyone is different and it is important for staff to get to know new residents and their families so they can provide the best and most meaningful care to them. When people move to residential care, staff assess their needs, likes and dislikes by talking with them and with their families (where appropriate). By asking a lot of questions they can find out more about new residents, including what is important to them. The questions may seem intrusive but it is important that the staff know as much about you as possible so they can tailor their care to your specific needs.

Staff are aware that the first few months after moving into residential care can be very challenging. They sometimes provide extra care and attention at this time to residents and their families. This may include becoming an advocate for a resident, building a relationship of trust with residents and their families, and maintaining regular follow-up to gauge how the resident is feeling in their new environment and community.

Increasingly, homes have pastoral care practitioners and staff who specialise in lifestyle activities (activities, hobbies, interests), and these staff can be very helpful in the settling in period. The pastoral care and lifestyle staff spend much of their time with residents and family members, helping them to feel comfortable in their new 'home', and with their fellow residents and care home staff. One experienced pastoral care practitioner described the role of pastoral care as, 'to bring everyone on the journey to the point of being comfortable where they are, emotionally, socially and psychologically'.

BERNADETTE'S STORY

Bernadette's story illustrates that you can embrace the change and be aware that your new home will be different, but that you don't have to sacrifice all that is important to you. You can be happy, more supported and still maintain independence in a care home.

Bernadette came to Australia as a young adult. Some of her family now live in Australia, too. Over the years, Bernadette has had several jobs and has remained independent, living alone and keeping up a rewarding social life. Since retirement, she has kept herself busy volunteering for charities and maintaining a close social network of family and friends, whom she catches up with regularly.

Now about 80 years of age, Bernadette says it had never occurred to her to move to residential care until her doctor made the suggestion. She was, however, aware that her health was not what it used to be, and that it seemed more difficult to get everything done, as she was not as energetic as she would like to be. At first, she was a bit confronted by her doctor's suggestion, thinking, 'Who, me? But I realised when he was talking, that I was in a bad situation. I wasn't able to look after myself.' And so, Bernadette did go and inspect the care home she is now living in. On reflection, Bernadette realises that she 'was not having great fun [living alone]' in the time leading up to her move to the care home. Furthermore, she no longer felt safe living alone. Soon after the talk with her doctor, Bernadette required respite in residential care. 'It was really good... I was so surprised!' she recalls. She started to think the doctor might be right and that moving to a care home permanently might make life better in many ways.

Now, although she needs reminding to register in the 'sign out' book for her regular outings, Bernadette has no complaints about having made the decision to move. She still loves going out and is happy that she is still able to do so. She is happy that there is a chapel at the home she lives at, too; she finds this very convenient – especially in the cold weather – and it enables her to maintain her spiritual life in the way she wishes to.

Bernadette still misses aspects of her 'old life' before her move. She commented that she misses the extra wardrobe space and the extra room she used to have. She has also found it hard to let go of treasured possessions, and remains surrounded by more of these than her room can easily accommodate – but she doesn't feel ready to let them go just yet. Bernadette does not, however, miss having to cook and shop and run a household. Furthermore, having a new community of people to connect with has, in her view, been a real bonus. And she feels that support from the staff and the pastoral care practitioners is right there if she needs it. In fact, the only big challenge she found since making her decision to move to residential care was how to manage the practical side of the move. When the pastoral care services team became aware of Bernadette's wish to move to a care home, they helped Bernadette arrange the move, and they continue to provide her with welcome support.

It has taken some months for Bernadette to feel she is 'home'. Initially after the move, Bernadette was telling herself periodically, 'I haven't got a home, now... I'm not doing anything positive,' then in an hour or so she would think, 'Don't be silly, you're doing well.' At this time, Bernadette noticed that she also had a sense of relief at being cared for, 'The people in charge were interested in (me), and the nurses, too, were marvellous... You had to convince yourself if you were going to go or going to stay, which I did, eventually.'

FROM THE PERSPECTIVE OF FAMILY AND FRIENDS – WHAT CAN HELP WITH THE SETTLING IN PROCESS?

Assuring the resident that they are still loved and not forgotten is probably the most important thing family and friends can do, and this is usually expressed by visiting them in their new home as much as possible. Spending time with your family member or friend can make a big difference to how well they adapt to living in residential care. More regular visits to the resident soon after transition to residential care may help them settle in.

Listening to the resident without interrupting them can help, as can engaging with the resident in an activity or a discussion that is meaningful to them. Personalising their room by displaying objects, family photographs and memorabilia that has special significance to the resident can also help, as long as it is done with the older person leading the changes. Taking the control of homely possessions away from their owner can lead to feelings of sadness and displacement as the person's identity that is tied up in their possessions is being taken away. Playing the resident's favourite music quietly can provide comfort if the person is in the mood for music, or they can listen to favourite programmes on the radio. Putting their favourite songs on an MP3 or audio player with headphones is a way to bring music that is personal and a favourite, familiar element back into the person's life. Residents can then listen to their favourite music in the lounge areas as well as their room.

With the older person's permission, bringing in 'treasured' possessions that hold special meaning and trigger memories for the resident can help them feel connected to their former life – and help others to learn about the resident's life, too. The timing for introduction of treasured possessions needs to be handled sensitively and it's important to follow the lead of the new resident. Another way of doing this is by assisting the resident to recall their memoirs, and for them to record these in a written, pictoral or digital form. Writing a description of the circumstances of each photograph on the back of each photo is a helpful prompt for staff and residents, too. Celebrating birthdays or other special occasions with your family member can also help. The care home staff can assist you with these processes.

Continuing to enjoy shared activities with the resident can make a positive difference. This may include outings from the care home, or activities at the care home, such as doing a jigsaw puzzle, playing cards, sorting objects, flower arranging, making a small garden or reminiscing about shared activities of the past.

Be aware that the new resident needs the time and gentle support to experience and move through this transition process and to adjust *at their own pace*. This is especially relevant if the resident is recently bereaved (including the loss of a spouse, friend or even a loved pet), and confronting a decline in their health, as well as having had to leave their old home.

During visits, ensuring your relative is given the opportunity to talk about how they are feeling can help them adjust to the care home. Organising a roster of visitors may work for some families and friendship groups connected to the resident, too, especially in the first few weeks after the resident moves in. Bringing in cherished pets for a visit to the new resident on a regular basis, or alternatively, providing photos of the resident's pet or access to other visiting pets, can help. For residents with significant cognitive impairment, something tactile like a soft blanket or shawl that smells or feels pleasant and familiar to them may help them to relax. Familiar or favourite smells provided through aromatherapy can also help. The smell of lavender oil has been shown to help with relaxation.

Introductions of the resident to other residents and staff by care staff can also help, although this may need to happen in stages after the move to residential care, depending on how the person is feeling. Some care homes assign a 'buddy' from staff to individual residents and encourage one of the existing residents to connect with a new person on a regular basis to prevent them feeling as though a sea of new faces has intruded into their everyday life. Ask the care home what their 'settling in' routine is for new residents and discuss how it can be tailored to help the individual.

Men can feel especially isolated when moving into a care home. A men's group was set up at one residence to provide a space in the care environment, which can often have far more females (residents and staff included) than males. The group gave the men an opportunity to have time with other men in an exclusively 'male' space that provided an extra avenue of support for them. For male partners living in care with their female partners with dementia, this can be especially supportive (see Chapter 8 on Diverse Needs).

Staff need to know what is important to you and your family members, so that you can continue to live your life, or your family member can live their life, in a way that is meaningful and respectful of their cultural practices, including any important routines and rituals. Discuss your needs with the staff and they will try and ensure that you are able to continue your important daily routines and practices.

FRANCINE AND GERARD'S STORY

Francine and Gerard's story illustrates that residents and family members should expect to be included in decision making, to be listened to and not to be rushed. For new residents, having a family member or a friend to support you soon after your move can be helpful, especially when talking about what your needs are with the staff.

Several months ago, Francine and her siblings assisted their father, Gerard, to move to a care home.

> The first few days were terribly difficult because he really felt that loss of independence. He really felt that. And we had a lot of, 'Well, Dad, you know, they're just getting to know you. Once they know you, you'll be able to do this, this, this and this.' That sort of thing. And, that's been true. Once they [staff] got to know him, that sort of dissipated... For us as a family, it was talking through, and letting Dad be able to vent, and, um, just talking him through it.

Gerard had lived independently in the family home for decades, and despite his increasing frailty, had continued to manage his finances, and to maintain his many social connections with friends, his large family and others in his local community. He also enjoyed his sport and other activities.

Unexpectedly, Gerard had a lengthy hospitalisation after a fall at his home. Gerard and his family had little time to adjust to the geriatrician's advice that he 'couldn't return home'. Eventually, all the family realised that it was necessary for Gerard to move, 'We were all on the same page in the end,' but the process of acceptance took some patience as well as 'emotionally charged' discussion among Francine and her siblings. Francine describes her father as 'stoic and accepting', when he heard he had to go to a care home. She reflects, 'It was so overwhelming for him. It was heartbreaking. But he listened... He knew what was going on.' Francine says that giving her father a continued sense of control of his life is very important:

> One piece of advice I would give people would be to include them [the family member going into aged care] in the process all along...and that was a very important thing for Dad, that he still had some control over that... He [Gerard] said, 'I just want to be kept informed. I just want to know what is going on.' So we've managed to do that all the way through.

There was little time to adjust, and quick decisions had to be made to secure a care home place that became available at a residence they had just become acquainted with. The family brought several things to help Gerard feel that the room was distinctively 'his'. They also organised for their father to have the telephone connected in his room, and for newspaper delivery, and they purchased a small fridge, to help him be 'a little bit more independent'. Since the move, Francine and her siblings have found the staff responsive to their requests and concerns:

We have only had one cause to complain... We consulted with him [Gerard] first...and they [management] have acted on it. Everyone is coming to him now, saying, 'Is that all right?' So, they did act on that. I think Dad felt pleased that something positive had come... I think that [sense of empowerment] is really important, when everything else is taken away from you.

Francine noted that her father, 'was never going to be one to get involved with the [frequent social] activities', and that it was important to him that he was not made to do things he did not enjoy. Gerard seems to have settled into his new home, according to his daughter; he has even learned that a couple of the residents have social links with his family, and he chats with them and other residents regularly. He also attends the communal dining room, goes to mass, has frequent visits from his family and 'old' friends, enjoys reading again, going out with his family and chatting on the telephone. Francine acknowledges that her father 'did not want to be there, so saying words like "enjoying it", we just sort of steered clear of those kind of words. He would not say, "It was the best thing that ever happened to me." He would say, "It's the right decision."'

Gerard has recently advised his friend, who is living alone in poor health that, 'You've got to come into a place like this, you know. You are looked after!' That is the kind of affirmation that he gives. 'He still calls the shots,' Francine comments.

HOW THE MOVING PROCESS FEELS FOR FAMILY AND FRIENDS

Getting and accepting support is very important, even if you and your family usually do not like to rely on others for help. At the time of transition to residential care, residents need support from their families and friends, and families and friends need support too. This support can come from a range of sources, including the care home staff and external organisations such as a counselling service, carer's association or older people's advocate organisation. It may include talking about the experience you are going through, and it may also include getting more information and resources that will help you know what to expect.

Helping to move a family member into residential care is often confronting for families. Families can feel as if they have abandoned their family member. This may be especially difficult where residential care placement is seen as 'breaking up the family' and where a family member has said, 'Never put me into a home.'

While there may be some positive aspects to the move to residential care for the resident, there will almost certainly be some negative aspects too. These are related to a sense of loss, enforced change and its accompanying sense of grief. For many people, it is the time they leave their family home, with its reminders of their lives up until now, their familiar neighbourhood sights and sounds, treasured neighbours and community, some friends and, maybe, their beloved pets.

From a family perspective, the family wants to know that someone is going to care for their relative as they would like to be looked after, and in the way that the family is familiar with. We know that family members are also experiencing many emotions, possibly including guilt, loss, grief and even a sense of relief when they help place a relative into residential care, relief that can trigger more guilt. Family members may also be feeling exhausted and stressed about the move. Pastoral care practitioners or counsellors may be available to talk to about the experience. Talking therapy can help families to learn some coping strategies for this new phase in their lives.

MERLE'S STORY

Merle's story illustrates that moving into residential care can be a smooth and happy transition for some people who feel they are ready to do so. Some prior planning, often with friends and family, can make the transition easier, and you do not have to lose your sense of independence in the process.

Merle has been living in residential aged care now for nearly 18 months. She had several children who kept her very busy, was widowed later in life, then she lived alone until her 90th year. Merle was not seriously considering residential care until her memory started to fail her more and more frequently. One day, Merle became lost when she went for a walk, and was unable to remember her name or where she lived. After this incident, she learned she had early stage Alzheimer's disease, and she decided she needed to move to a care home: 'I was quite happy to go somewhere,' she recalls. Merle had sometime earlier discussed with a friend 'where we would go next...we weren't that serious, but we broached the subject [of future residential care]... We'd decided to go together.' She informed her family of her decision, and she remembered the care home her friend had considered sometime before as, 'good... if [they] ever needed to go into care'. As it happened, her friend did eventually join her at the same care home. This has helped make Merle's transition to residential care relatively easy; she and her friend spend many happy hours together, even if they do miss being able to go out to the shops for a cup of coffee together. In addition, Merle has a supportive family who helped her pack up her old home, and who keep in frequent contact with her. She also goes out regularly with some of them.

Merle went to boarding school and she remembers arriving at the care home, being shown her room and feeling as if she had been transported back to school, 'They even had a bell to tell you when it was lunchtime,' she recalls. The set-up seemed strangely familiar, although she comments that she can make far more decisions for herself now, living in residential care, than she could at school. This thought makes her laugh out loud, and her eyes crinkle at the corners as she smiles and reflects on her move.

Even before she was married, Merle lived independently and remained independent when she was married, 'I've always done my own thing... I'm me and I don't have a whole lot of people telling me what to do.' Merle was comfortable making her own decisions, so moving to a residence that treated her as a person capable of making decisions was very important to her. She says she feels she has a lot of freedom to do what she wishes in her new home – except go shopping on her own. Merle cannot recall visiting the care home before she moved in, she may have, she says, but what was important to her was that she made the decision to go herself, and she felt relaxed going to this particular home that she had already heard about and discussed with her friend.

CHAPTER 5

RESILIENCE AND ADJUSTING TO CHANGE

THE ROLLER COASTER OF CHANGE

From the perspective of the older person moving into residential care, expect that adjusting to a new home will take some time, but there are ways to assist with the settling-in process. Everyone copes with change differently, and it is normal to feel that a change brings conflicting emotions to the fore. Ellis (2010) and Fisher (2000) discussed nine stages of transition that people can go through in adjusting to a big change such as moving into care (see Table 5.1).

Table 5.1: Stages in adjusting to change associated with moving into care

Anxiety – anxiety associated with moving into care is brought about by not knowing what the future will be like, and whether the person will be able to enjoy their new situation.
Happiness – positive feelings associated with the change can be due to a feeling that things will improve, that the person will be experiencing better care than before.
Fear – fear of having to learn new things, new interactions and acting in a new way are all common responses.

cont.

Threat – a major lifestyle change can be perceived as threatening. People may be unclear about what is going to happen, may fear that control is being taken away from them, and the control is handed to someone whom the person does not trust to act in their best interests.
Guilt – the older person may feel guilty that they have not been able to cope alone, that they are causing difficulties for other people, or spending money that could have been used by their relatives or for a different purpose.
Depression – feelings of low self-esteem, lack of motivation and confusion are associated with the loss and grief some people feel as they let go of their previous lifestyle, and perhaps let go of a vision for their future that is no longer possible. People may lose their sense of identity, who they thought they were, and fear taking on the new identity of 'someone who lives in a care home'.
Disillusionment – some people may feel that their values, goals and beliefs are not the same as those around them, as either their family may be pressuring them to move, or their doctor has advised them to move into care. This may lead to withdrawal from those around them as the person no longer feels engaged or in tune with those around them.
Hostility – some people may express their feelings as hostility, angry that the situation is different to what they expected. Sometimes grief can be expressed as hostility, or anger may be a lifelong response to situations where the person has lost control or disagrees with events.
Denial – it can be difficult to accept any change, and sometimes people may deny that the change will occur and keep denying the change even after moving into care, ignoring evidence to the contrary.
Complacency – there may be a final stage of emotions, having survived the change and worked through all the emotional stages above, some people emerge feeling as though they are operating once again within their comfort zone.

Adapted from Ellis (2010)

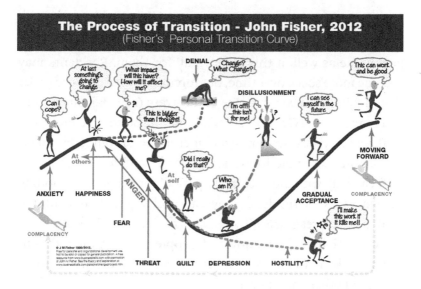

Figure 5.1: The process of transition according to John Fisher (2012)

Reproduced with permission from John Fisher

How people settle in to a care home varies from person to person. The first few months can be the most difficult time for people transitioning to residential care. People with less family support or with cognitive impairment can be more vulnerable and require extra care. They may ask when they are 'going home', and they may want to pack their bags or ask for your assistance to do so, or be forlornly waiting at the door when you leave or arrive at the care home. This can be very upsetting for the resident and their family, and the staff are trained to support you at such times.

How easily residents make the transition and feel 'settled' can depend not only on lifelong coping strategies but also on what the resident's life circumstances are, how much they enjoy socialising and how much support they have.

Some residents may not have been very social before admission, and may prefer to minimise social contact in their new home as well, if this is 'normal' for them. Residents may become more social over time, but forcing them to be more social than they wish to be can cause them stress (see Malcolm's story, and Francine and Gerard's story). It may be better to consult the staff, and to visit your family member in their room for a while.

Pastoral care practitioners, care staff and lifestyle activities staff can help with the 'settling in period' for residents by finding out what it is the resident enjoys, and helping them to continue with these interests, if at all possible. They may also be introduced to new activities they enjoy and people they get on with, but some residents will need more time to adjust and be ready to do this – and others may never wish to.

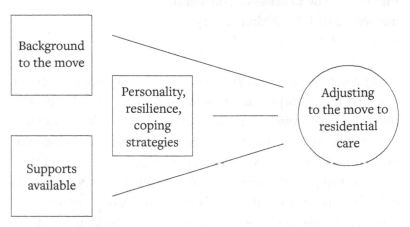

Figure 5.2: Factors that affect how long it takes to adjust to living in a care home

Many residents say they feel happier about being in residential care than remaining in their own home. If they are now feeling less lonely and more supported with their daily activities in residential care than they were at home, they can feel settled more quickly. It is unusual for people not to adjust, and some people can adjust within a few months. Personal resilience will play a big part, as will the degree to which a resident feels they were involved in the choice to move to residential care, and the amount of trusted support they receive.

It is hard to generalise, but residents who are 'settling in' can be seen to take themselves off to activities more readily and become more involved with what is happening at the care home, and connect more with other residents, rather than staying in their room alone.

For the family carer, the transition to a new lifestyle can take time to adjust to as well. Research studies have found that some family carers are still adjusting to the new care arrangements some time after the move as they continue to process the emotions associated with the change.

Resilience is a psychological term that is used often in describing children's adjustment to stresses, but less so for older people and their families. The individual's resilience in adjusting to the change encountered with moving to residential care is part of their personality. According to the American Psychological Association (APA), resilience is 'the process of adapting well in the face of adversity, trauma, tragedy, threats or significant sources of stress – such as family and relationship problems or workplace and financial stressors. It means "bouncing back" from difficult experiences' (American Psychological Association 2017). Being resilient does not mean that the experience is not difficult for the person, but rather that they draw on their own resources to help them to adjust. According to the APA, there are ways resilience can be encouraged (see below).

Ways to build resilience

Make connections – with friends or family. Find someone who can listen or just be with you during times of stress. If there is no one in your family or friends, then someone in the care home may be there for you, if there is a pastoral care worker, or a volunteer. Some homes have befriending volunteers who can help you to feel that you are not alone.

Change the way you think about it – think about how the future will be better, and the current stress will pass. Watch out for any feelings that are signs that you are feeling a little better and focus on those rather than on the difficulties.

Accept that nothing ever stays the same – change is part of living, and nothing will stay the same, no matter where you live. Accepting that circumstances have changed will allow you to move on. Focus on the things you can change, however small, rather than the things you cannot change.

Have some goals – do something regularly even if just a small accomplishment that can give you a positive view of how the day has gone. Ask yourself, 'What is one thing I can accomplish today that helps me adjust to my new surroundings?'

Face your fears – take decisive action about a problem that is really bothering you, rather than detaching yourself and wishing it would go away. If something that the staff do is really upsetting you, take courage and speak up about it to try to improve it.

Look for opportunities for self-discovery – people often discover new depths as a result of a loss, and can become stronger with a heightened sense of their own spirituality and greater appreciation for life.

Nurture yourself – give yourself time to adjust, and allow yourself to have good days and bad days without castigating yourself that you are not coping. Take care of yourself by relaxing and looking out for activities that you enjoy, even simple pleasures such as enjoying a flower in bloom or a sunny day.

Avoid thinking it is a catastrophe – try to keep things in perspective, and keep a longer-term perspective. Even a painful health issue will not stay the same, and in the future you will not feel the same all the time, some days will be better than others.

Stay optimistic – expect that good things will happen. Try thinking about the good things and look forward to pleasant events rather than worrying about the things that you fear.

Adapted with permission from www.apa.org/helpcenter/road-resilience.aspx
Copyright © 2017 American Psychological Society

If a person has made the decision themselves to move, it can be an easier transition. Over time, a person may have lost their long-term social support networks in the community. Furthermore, someone being admitted from rehabilitation or after respite may have had the time to consider whether residential care can give them the support they need. For these people, the sense of new-found companionship and community, and the support that accompanies a residential care lifestyle, can be most welcome. Some new residents occasionally meet existing residents whom they knew years before, which can enrich their time in a care home.

Where the move to residential care has been made without the opportunity to prepare for the move, transition can be especially difficult. This can occur where a person has moved directly from hospital after a health care crisis, when you or your family member expected to go back home. Most people who are able to plan for and be involved in decision making for their move to residential care find it a helpful process that enables them to adapt to the change.

The sudden change of routine and environment that accompanies a move to residential care can still be difficult though, even for those who are more resolved about the move. Simple things can remind you or your family member of how things have changed. Having to live with others when you are used to living alone, or living with people you have not chosen to live with, is understandably challenging for new residents. For residents who do not have a cognitive impairment, it may be confronting to live with other residents who do.

It is important to remember that the move can trigger a sense of grief associated with losses, and residents may lose confidence for a while, or may experience a period of depression during the transition period. With time and appropriate care, however, most people do adjust to residential care and to their new community.

BRENDA'S STORY

Brenda's story illustrates that thinking about the possibility of moving to residential care, and discussing this with family or friends, can make it easier to identify what sort of care would suit you best. Then, if a time comes when you need care, you and your family may find the transition smoother. Making new friends can also help a lot after you move to a care home.

Brenda lived independently in a retirement village for many years. She had spent much of her working life caring for others, including some family members, before her move to the village several years ago. She soon established enduring friendships with her local community.

Eighteen months ago, prompted by a health crisis requiring hospitalisation, Brenda decided to move again, this time, to a care home, as she was left feeling vulnerable and uncomfortable about living alone. On reflection, Brenda thinks that subconsciously she was preparing for a time when she might need to move to residential care; she had even discussed the move with a close friend. She says that the decision was timely for her, 'I didn't let it go too long, get too sick, when I couldn't absorb what was going on.'

Brenda has a supportive extended family and states that she did not feel pressured by them in any way to move. 'I'd heard such good reports about this place,' she says. The care home was situated conveniently for her and her family, so they could continue to visit Brenda frequently. Brenda visited the home with some of her family members and was very impressed: 'Right from the very beginning, I took to it...[my family] took me to see the residence before I moved in. And even that day, I felt at home.'

Despite Brenda making the decision to move voluntarily and unhurriedly, it was still difficult leaving the community that she had been so attached to. 'Moving after [many] years was a big wrench... perhaps more emotionally,' she comments.

Brenda's family assisted her in packing up her house, and she has some favourite pieces of furniture in her room, which faces the garden and a birdbath. The latter gives her much joy as she watches a variety of birds come and go during the day. Brenda also enjoys her puzzles and attending the regular exercise classes with her friend, Lois. The mutual support and company Brenda and Lois provide to one another has made living at the care home an even happier choice for Brenda. 'Having company has made a big difference, it's helped a lot,' she says. 'We do have fun.' Brenda identifies the social contact she has had as crucial in helping her adjust to living in a care home. The proximity to the local church and regular opportunities to attend mass have also been important for Brenda. In addition, she emphasises that she enjoys the food. 'My only complaint is there is too much,' she says.

Brenda states that she has found the transition to a care home easier than she expected. Soon after she moved into the residence, she met the pastoral care practitioner, 'who introduced herself, explained who she was and what her work was'. Brenda has since developed a friendship with the pastoral care practitioner, who she says supports her and cares for her. Brenda comments that all the staff are, 'so, so kind – even if you are not sick...nothing's a hassle for them. I have been overwhelmed with the kindness here.'

CHAPTER 6

HOW TO MAINTAIN PURPOSE IN LIFE

Your interests, likes, dislikes; it is all still there [when you are older].

PASTORAL CARE PRACTITIONER

The French have a phrase *'raison d'etre'* or 'reason for being'. The Japanese have a word for 'reason for being' – *ikigai* – a combination of 'iki', meaning life, and 'kai', meaning what one expects and hopes for. Everyone has a reason for being, and it is worthwhile to reflect on what is most important to you when moving into residential care. What is it that helps you to get up in the morning, in a spiritual sense? In middle age, people may consider their purpose in life is to earn enough income to pay the bills, or to bring their children up, and in retirement many people struggle to maintain a sense of purpose for their lives. They may continue a life of service by volunteering or helping to care for grandchildren, or devote their lives to further learning or exploring the world. A sense of purpose is something that is needed, regardless of the stage of life. One study of the association between sense of purpose and health outcomes for a large sample (43,319) of Japanese people found that the group who believed that their life was worth living had a lower rate of cardiovascular disease and had a lower mortality rate than the group who were without this belief (Sone *et al.* 2008).

How can people moving into care homes maintain their sense of purpose in life? To find your reason for being you may need to do some reflecting and some self-searching. After moving to residential care, you should try to continue with whatever activities used to provide you with fulfilment, purpose and meaning. This may be gardening, listening to the radio, reading, keeping connected to current affairs, walking, regular access to cherished pets or continuing to enjoy another activity that gives you pleasure, such as craft or physical activities, discussion groups, singing, music, dancing, laughter, painting, time chatting (with friends, other residents and their families) watching sport or movies, playing scrabble or reading. The list is endless – the main message is to maintain some interest. Maintaining interest may mean accepting that the way the interest is followed has to change – watching sport on television rather than attending in person, or listening to a gardening programme on the radio rather than weeding. And remember that taking up a new hobby or interest can be invigorating and good for brain health at any age.

For some residents, being introduced to others who are interested in similar things is most welcome, and can help them feel as if they are 'settling in'. For others, having the opportunity to be alone and enjoy some privacy might be very important to help them adjust to the many changes happening in their lives and to give them time to reflect quietly. Staff should understand the importance of being aware of what each new resident may need in terms of social connection or space, and that needs can change.

Some new residents find that attending a faith-sharing group, either at the care home, or externally in the local community, helps them to feel purposeful and connected, as might religious residents attending religious ceremonies. The staff, including the lifestyle and pastoral care staff, try to identify the interests of residents so that they can help link them with others who have similar interests, or set up new groups for residents based on mutual interests. Any information that you or your family member provide that helps staff get to know you better as a person will enable the care home to provide the best care, including the opportunity to engage in activities you or your family member like. Visiting family members may also wish to be included in some of these activities.

Residents often tell us that they want to 'contribute to their community in a useful way'. This might mean assisting in regular daily activities at the care home that make them feel 'at home', such as arranging flowers, tidying, sorting or making something, or it might mean residents connecting with the external community, such as making gifts to sell for charity groups in the community.

Residents should feel free to discuss with senior staff what it is that they need to find meaning and purpose in life. Staff should also check with residents to see how they can improve residents' care and quality of life, so that they feel valued and respected.

Often in care homes there will be staff whose main work is to provide interesting and fun activities that engage residents and give them purpose. As a resident, choose activities that suit your life purpose, that you enjoy and that will help you to feel as though your life has meaning. Ask staff for help to allow you to engage with other activities if your interests are not on offer. Not all activities will suit everyone, some will seem lacking in purpose or just provided for filling time. Take note of how the activity makes you feel and only choose to participate in activities that really suit you. These are the ones that will give you joy and make you feel 'happy to be alive'. When you are adjusting to residential care, you may be inclined not to participate in anything at all. If this feeling persists for longer than a few months and you feel as though you have lost interest in previous interests, it may be a symptom of depression. It is important to discuss this with care staff who can help to improve things for you.

Table 6.1: Life with meaning – what makes us 'happy to be alive'?

Which type of activity in the list below makes you happy to be alive? What is most important to you to give your life meaning? Tick if this applies to you, and think of an event or activity that you could include in your day. Show the care home staff or discuss with them what they might be able to make happen in your day

Type of activity that helps me feel happy to be alive	Example	Tick
Freedom, adventure and feeling involved in the world	An outing to a public event	
Love for and connections to others	A visit, phone call or memory photo album	
Expressing myself, sharing my thoughts and offering my wisdom	Giving a talk, discussing a topic I am interested in	
Experiencing things that are pleasurable to my senses	Listening to a music concert, or having a massage	
Belonging to a group/ community	Joining a club or group activity offered in the care home	
Being competitive, working on my own or in a team towards winning	Playing bridge or a card game	
Challenging my mind, being interested in things and learning	Doing a jigsaw puzzle, hearing a talk from an expert	
Being devoted to a higher power, for example my faith, spirituality	Taking part in a religious ceremony	
Being creative, achieving and or contributing towards something	Making art or woodwork or gardening	
Being fit, healthy and independent	Taking part in an exercise group	

Having fun and being able to relax and unwind	Joining in a Friday drinks social, watching a show or dancing	
Being of service to others, giving and helping where I can	Helping a resident who is less able than I am	

Adapted with permission from Brownfield (2017) Better Practice Conference Melbourne 2017 and Vasey RSL Care

STEPHEN AND MAEVE'S STORY

Stephen and Maeve's story illustrates that it can take some time to adjust to the new way of life that is living in residential care.

After many years living together and raising several children, Stephen and Maeve, both aged in their 80s, had some hard decisions to make. Maeve had a medical condition affecting her mobility. This made it increasingly difficult for her to stay at home with Stephen as her main carer. After being hospitalised, the couple reluctantly agreed that Maeve would best receive the care she needed in the care home her daughter had located. Stephen described the move from the family home as 'A dramatic change. A bit traumatic, knowing if you have done the right thing. I came every day to see her [to visit Maeve at the care home].'

Stephen also had health issues, and about a year after Maeve's move, and after a discussion with his children, Stephen thought, 'Life is short, I better get in there,' and decided to join Maeve at the same care home.

Stephen considers that the care home is beautifully situated, reflecting that, 'When we walked in the front door, you could tell it was a bit different.' Maeve adds, 'You could walk from one end of the place to the other.' This was important to them, as both have issues with walking.

The couple originally shared a room at the care home, but they no longer do for practical reasons. Their rooms are, however, close, and they spend their days together watching television, reading, attending exercise classes and group games, and doing puzzles. Occasionally, they go out for a meal with their family, which they really enjoy. They have social interaction with staff, too, whom they find very supportive.

Stephen comments that they both feel that they have 'reasonable freedom' to do as they wish in the care home, despite the restrictions imposed by their health. Stephen says it took about six months for him to adjust to residential care. Initially, he needed a lot more structure because he was used to organising his days to be quite full. Now, he says, he has learned to 'go with the flow' and not plan each day in such a structured way, and he feels more relaxed, quipping, 'Thank God I've got all day to do this.'

It also took Maeve 'about six months' for the care home to feel like 'home', and she described feeling 'looked after' from the moment she first arrived. Maeve added that having her friends visit her regularly when she first moved really helped her feel more settled, as did attending regular mass and receiving visits from the pastoral care practitioner. These activities also provide her and Stephen with the opportunity to meet more of their neighbours at the residence.

Maeve's room is very home-like and the couple seem most comfortable sharing the space. The couple say it is a smallish space to share during the day, but they think the arrangement works well for them and they both enjoy looking out at the garden.

When Stephen first heard of couples in residential care living in separate rooms, he said he thought, 'Hell, what a stupid idea! But now, in here, I am inclined to think, well, you haven't complained really [directed at Maeve, who smiles].'

CHAPTER 7

LIVING WITH DEMENTIA IN A CARE HOME

M any older people living in care homes have dementia, which causes memory loss or thinking impairment. Moving house can be especially confusing for someone with these issues. Dementia is a progressive disease, and often professionals will recommend moving to a safer environment as the disease gets worse. How can we make this move as comfortable as possible for the individual with dementia and their family? And for people without dementia, what is it like to start living with people who do have dementia? This chapter provides some basic information about what dementia is, and how moving into residential care can affect someone with dementia. It also discusses what it is like living with someone with dementia for those who may be physically frail but mentally alert.

WHAT IS DEMENTIA?

Dementia is a term that refers to a range of symptoms associated with a decline in memory and thinking ability, severe enough to cause the person experiencing dementia to have difficulty in performing everyday activities. While memory and some types of thinking can decline gradually with age, the type of cognitive impairment associated with dementia is of a different level to normal age-related memory decline.

Dementia is not a single disease. It is an umbrella term for a group of symptoms that can be caused by a number of different diseases. Alzheimer's disease is one type of dementia. There are other diseases that are associated with changes in thinking and memory ability and ability to care for yourself. Alzheimer's disease is the most well-known form of dementia, and also the most common, accounting for 50–70 per cent of all cases. Other types of dementia are vascular dementia and Lewy body dementia. Some people with Parkinson's disease develop a type of dementia, and other less common types of dementia such as Pick's disease and dementia associated with HIV (human immunodeficiency virus) are also part of this group of diseases that have in common some deterioration in memory and thinking ability that interferes with everyday functioning.

The symptoms of dementia are varied, but the symptom that most people are familiar with is memory loss. Not everyone with dementia experiences memory loss, depending on the parts of the brain that are not working properly. We all have days when we feel as though our brain is not working as well as it should, but the cognitive changes associated with dementia are persistent and progressive. While we may forget where we put the car keys, a person with dementia may forget what the car keys are for as well. Short-term memory may be more impaired than memory for things that happened a long time ago. The impairment can cause people to forget how to do daily routine tasks such as boiling the kettle, making a cup of tea or getting dressed.

Dementia can happen to anyone, but there is increasing research about what the risk factors are for developing dementia and importantly how or whether dementia can be prevented by taking certain actions. So far, we know that age is still the biggest risk factor for developing dementia. As you get older, your chances increase for developing dementia. For people aged 70–74, about one in 30 people will develop dementia, but among those over 90 years of age, about one in three people will have dementia. Rarely, people develop dementia at younger ages, and there are cases of people in their 30s, 40s or 50s developing dementia (in the UK around 5 per cent of people with dementia are under 65).

Some people with dementia have no family history at all of the disease and there is evidence that some types of dementia are associated with genetic risk factors. About one-third of people with Alzheimer's disease have a close relative who had dementia. This is not to say that if you have a relative with dementia then you will also definitely develop dementia, but it increases your risk of developing it.

Dementia affects people in different ways. It can start with small changes in personality or behaviour. Some people start to lose the ability to initiate activities, which can be interpreted as depression, or there may be other subtle changes in personality. Some partners may interpret these changes as a sign that the individual wants to leave their marriage as they begin to withdraw or change responses to their partner. When the speech area of the brain is affected, people start to lose the ability to find the right word in conversation, or they may start to repeat themselves as memory loss interferes with everyday conversational ability. The individual may experience mood changes, accompanying the confusion and anxiety. These mood changes can be in response to the individual realising that their abilities are declining, or the changes may be due to changes in the brain associated with the disease.

Family and friends can play a big part in assisting the older person with dementia to cope with the disease. Family can be a link to the past for the person, as they can provide prompts to events that are important in the person's life. Receiving reassurance from family and friends that the person is still loved and is still considered as the same person, despite some changes, can help to maintain the person's identity. It can be very challenging for family and friends to stay connected with the person with dementia, especially when personality changes make it seem as though the individual is no longer the person they used to be. Dementia can change some core aspects of an individual. Someone who was once demure and polite may seem rude as they lose the executive control in their brain that once stopped them from saying certain things. Families and friends can find these changes especially heartbreaking as they feel a loss of the person they used to know, without actually being able to mourn the person's death. Some people are embarrassed or frightened by the changes associated with dementia, and may avoid social situations in case the person with dementia does or says something that they feel ashamed of. Some cultural groups find dementia symptoms especially difficult, as deteriorating mental health can hold a particularly strong stigma in some cultures.

Unfortunately, there is no cure for dementia, although the scientific community is working hard to find one. Some medications have been found to relieve some of the symptoms for short periods of time, but individual responses are quite varied so medical supervision is important. Now clinical guidelines recommend that behavioural and psychological symptoms of dementia can be addressed with psychological treatments and changes to the environment that can help the person with dementia and their carers to cope with daily living.

Alzheimer's Australia recommend that family and friends can help someone with dementia in the following ways

- Learn as much as you can about dementia. Local Alzheimer's associations run education groups, and there are many free resources available online as well. Make sure the online resource is endorsed by an authority such as the Alzheimer's Association or local medical authority.

- Look after yourself by scheduling regular breaks from caring, and maintaining your own social supports.
- Be available for a chat with the person with dementia, without being in a hurry.
- Bring a meal, or help with gardening or shopping.
- Support the person with dementia to continue with some of the things they enjoyed doing before their diagnosis. Sometimes they may need modification, for example, watching the football on TV together instead of actually going to the game.
- Remember that people with dementia can still enjoy the moment, even if it is forgotten soon after.
- Ask the person with dementia how you can help.

Adapted from Alzheimer's Australia (2005)

COMMUNICATING WITH SOMEONE WITH DEMENTIA

Someone with dementia may find the move to residential care especially difficult if they have not been involved in the decision making process. The Alzheimer's Association in the USA recommends that being honest and providing as much information as possible is still appropriate, even for someone with memory loss. Writing some things down can help, as people with dementia can retain reading ability while their ability to understand the spoken word is deteriorating. Some people with dementia can have a mixture of hearing impairment and cognitive or thinking impairment, so the combination can make conversation difficult. Some changes, such as difficulty in finding the right word or inability to understand what you are saying, can make communication challenging. The use of photographs in certain contexts may be helpful to prompt memory for people living with dementia.

Table 7.1: Points to remember when communicating with someone with dementia

Be positive and agreeable, focusing on what the person can do – try not to be condescending or to remind the person that they do not remember things well
Distraction and diversion are good tools – arguing, blocking or shaming are not helpful for anyone
Reminiscing about how the situation was handled in the past can help
Modeling with body language and facial expression can take the anxiety out of a situation
Encouraging with positive reinforcement or praise rather than forcing will lead to a better outcome

Adapted from http://alzheimersadvocate.com/caregiver-help/poster

Researchers have found that communication consists of three factors: the words that are being spoken, the tone of voice and our body language, which is the way our body is held while communicating, our facial expression, our posture, including the way our arms and hands are held. According to Albert Mehrabian, an American psychologist, non-verbal communication conveys far more than the words we are speaking when we are speaking about feelings and attitudes (Mehrabian 1981). Body language is thought to account for more than half (55 per cent) of communication. His model of communication showed that only 7 per cent of what we communicate verbally is the content of the message. The tone and pitch of our voice are thought to account for 38 per cent of what is communicated. So, according to this model, the words we use are only a small part of communication when talking about feelings or attitudes. This is illustrated in Figure 7.1, which shows that body language communicates far more than words.

This can be an advantage and disadvantage for communicating with someone with dementia about moving into residential care, as the person may not understand the words you are saying. When speaking with someone with dementia, it will help if you remain calm and speak in a gentle way. Keep background noise to a minimum to avoid distraction. Sitting in a quiet space will help the person with dementia to understand what you are saying. Holding their hand, keeping still and making eye contact will help to get the message across. Try to keep sentences short and simple – this is harder than it sounds as it is difficult to change the habits of a lifetime of speaking.

Talking about feelings and attitudes according to the Mehrabian model of communication

Body language

Tone and pitch of voice

Words

Figure 7.1: Illustrating that words are only a small part of what is communicated

What will not help is arguing and giving orders to the person with dementia. This style of communication is upsetting for anyone.

Instead, try to emphasise what the person with dementia can still do, rather than what they are no longer able to do.

WHAT IS THE IMPACT ON FAMILY CARERS?

For the carer of someone with dementia, the transition into residential care is an extra transition – they are already experiencing a transition associated with the condition of dementia. The person with dementia experiences changes in memory ability, communication ability, thinking ability and ability to do basic activities of daily living. On top of constant change for the person with dementia and their carer, yet another change associated with a new living arrangement is understandably a big adjustment. By the time someone with dementia moves into residential care, their family carer can be exhausted from the effort of caring and the stress of finding a residential care place as well as organising and negotiating for the transition to care for their family member. The person with dementia may be in the mid to late stages of dementia and not be able to understand or remember why they are moving. For their carer, the move may feel like another loss, and some carers report that the move into residential care is associated with a grief reaction. Often carers start to think about residential care when they are exhausted and feel as though they are no longer able to provide a good quality of care.

The reasons for thinking about residential care that are expressed by carers in research studies include: the need to improve safety for the person with dementia and for themselves; being unable to cope with the behaviours that the person with dementia has started to show; feelings of being trapped by the carer role; and feeling exhausted, physically or emotionally (Brown 2012). Arguably, family carers would be well placed to start preparing for a possible move into residential care earlier in the journey of caring, before they get to the stage of exhaustion but this means negotiating a well of feelings and emotions, which can also use energy. Ultimately, giving some thought to how the future might be handled would be very helpful for carers, and also for their family member.

The decision to move may have positive and negative emotions – positive, that the person will be cared for 24 hours a day and be safe, perhaps safer than they would have been living in the community. These feelings of relief are associated with the decision to move having finally been made; the person is safe and the responsibility of 24-hour care is now being shared with the care home. Yet they can be tinged with guilt as well, as carers wonder whether the choice of home is the best that can be made, and the carer has to adjust to loss of their own role as the main carer. The move has now left a gap in the carer's life. For a carer who is the person's spouse, the move can be especially difficult as they may have lived together for many years and are now facing what feels like a separation or the end of their marital life. Research has shown that many carers feel 'rushed' by the decision-making process. There are many aspects of the move to consider all at once, so the 'rushed' feeling is associated with having to process so many different considerations. It has been identified that there are five stages of grief and loss associated with being a carer of someone with dementia (Brown 2012): loss felt at the time of diagnosis initially, then again as the personality of the person with dementia begins to change; then again when the person moves to residential care; then again during palliative care and at the time of death; and again as the carer loses their identity as 'carer' and begins to take on other identities. At each of these stages of loss some accommodation and processing have to be made to adjust to the new situation and to focus on the future (see the discussion on resilience in Chapter 5).

WHAT IS THE IMPACT OF CHANGE LIKELY TO BE FOR PEOPLE WITH DEMENTIA?

As with people without cognitive impairment, many people with dementia are reluctant to move away from their family home. More research is required about how best to support people who have cognitive impairment in a care home environment, and to help them transition well to this care. Some research has shown that moving can be associated with good outcomes. There can be improved emotional well-being with the extra support that comes with residential care, better awareness of the environment if there is tailoring for people with dementia that may not have been possible in the family home, more participation in activities such as social groups (Aminzadeh *et al.* 2009).

However, there have been other studies showing that people with dementia fare poorly with the transition and experience depression, loneliness and a decline in functioning. This individual variability in the response to moving into care can be expected, as there are so many factors that vary from one individual's circumstances to another. Factors such as how well the person was functioning before they moved into care, lifelong personality traits and ways of coping, and the circumstances of the move will all play a part in determining how the transition goes. If the person has emotional support available before and during the transition, then that may influence how well the transition is accepted. How the care home responds to the individual will also determine how well they adjust to the change, so the responsibility for adjustment does not only lie with the individual and their family – it is a team effort. There are some things we do know: most people seem to respond positively to special attention and the chance to chat – whether or not they have a cognitive impairment. Calm spaces are known to help soothe people with a cognitive impairment, as do clear signs and reminders of where they are and what day it is. As one pastoral care practitioner said, it is a case of 'just meeting with this person where they are at, and making their day', by acknowledging them and connecting with them.

WHAT HELPS PEOPLE WITH DEMENTIA OR COGNITIVE IMPAIRMENT ADJUST TO CHANGE?

Introducing your relative with dementia or cognitive impairment gradually to the care home before they are moved there permanently can help some people. Visiting at least once or twice, briefly, will introduce some familiarity, even if they are unable to retrieve a memory of it. People who have used respite care before they move to residential care have reported that they were happy to move to the home as the respite care went well. Using respite care as a transition to permanent care can ease the adjustment for both the family and for the person with dementia.

The way the move occurs can have a big impact on the adjustment process. Family carers need some support with practical aspects of the move, for example, help to manage the paperwork involved as well as support with adjusting to the emotional aspects. There are many sources of information and checklists available for carers undergoing this stage (some are shown in Appendix 1 of this book).

When the person with dementia moves, the care home can provide an orientation programme and a welcome for the new resident. The family can ask the new carers how they will handle the first day, what will happen and how the new resident will be made to feel at home, to give them an idea of how the process will occur and to help them to prepare the new resident for the experience. An orientation pack for the person moving and one for their family can help, as it is hard to remember all the new information being provided. Some homes offer a 'buddy' so that a particular staff member and/or a particular resident are assigned to a new resident to help them feel as though there is a familiar face in the home.

The person with dementia can be included in decision making to help them feel as though they have control and are not being excluded from the conversation. Spending time with the person with dementia and discussing with them the reasons for moving, including how the experience is affecting the family carer as well, can help to keep the lines of communication open.

Preparation for residential care can be problematic for people with cognitive impairment and memory problems. People with dementia may forget that they have been involved in decision making about the move to residential care; this is difficult for the family members and can cause confusion and distress if residents believe they have been 'forced' to move. People with a cognitive impairment such as dementia can find any sort of change in routine unsettling, so a move to a care home may mean they seem 'not themselves' for a time, until they can adjust.

On a practical level, ensuring your relative living with dementia has familiar objects, sounds and smells can be calming. Having a large easy-to-read calendar in their room can help, so you can write appointments down, and mark off the days you have been to visit. Clearly labelling your relative's clothes and all other personal belongings, so they know what is theirs, can also help. Some care homes may provide a labelling service. For someone with dementia, the settling in period can be a confusing time. They can feel lonely and disoriented if they have forgotten why their family carer is not there. The emotional response for the person with dementia can be as strong as that of the family carer. After moving in, the person with dementia may continuously ask staff if they can go home, reflecting their anxiety that they are in a place where they do not feel relaxed and which does not feel like home.

If you are unsure of what to do or what might help you or your relative, seek the advice and support of staff to help you.

Most people with dementia do well when moving into residential care. While initially there may be some change in the behaviours exhibited as they adjust to their new surroundings, there will be positives associated with the move. Living in the company of others will suit many people. The staff will know how to respond to someone with dementia, and some homes will have special training for staff to learn how to support someone with memory loss. When choosing a care home, it is worth asking a care home manager about the type of training their staff receive, especially when your family member has dementia. Some aspects of dementia that were especially challenging living at home will be easier to manage with 24-hour care. For example, staff will be able to respond to changes in biorhythm such as night-time wakening more easily than family carers who may have been exhausted by sleep disturbances.

IS A SPECIAL CARE UNIT BETTER FOR PEOPLE WITH DEMENTIA?

Many family members and care home staff consider that separating people with dementia into separate, segregated accommodation is better for people with dementia than having people with and without dementia sharing the same communal living. Older people without dementia may find that separate arrangements suit them as they do not have to worry about intrusive or upsetting behaviour from fellow residents with cognitive impairment. Some care homes provide a special dementia unit, where there are different staffing levels, different activities offered and an environment that is quieter than the average communal lounge area. There has been a great deal of research conducted in this area, but no firm conclusions have yet been made, partly because there are so many factors that vary from one care home to the next that it is impossible to generalise.

Increasingly, care homes with special units are opening the doors and allowing people with dementia to move freely from one area to the next, without any detrimental effect. It is becoming clearer that training in dementia care is vital for staff so that staff understand how to prevent agitation in residents with dementia. A promising approach that is an alternative to a segregrated area is based on the Montessori model, which was originally developed for early childhood education by Maria Montessori, whereby people with dementia are offered structured activities intensively throughout the day in a separate area of the care home, akin to walking to a day care area, after which they return to their own room, which may or may not be in the same area of the care home. This type of person-centred care can be offered regardless of whether there is a locked door separating residents. Homes with smaller units where residents can get to know each other work well, and having staff who are trained in dementia care is perhaps more important than having a separate physical environment. We know that some physical environments can be confusing for people with dementia, and that signage, colours and spaces can help people with dementia to enjoy their environment.

HOW TO HANDLE THE VISIT TO A FAMILY MEMBER WITH DEMENTIA

Visiting a family member in their new surroundings can be upsetting for everyone concerned. It may be hard to know what to do during the visit, how to respond to questions about going home and how to spend the time visiting. For the family member, it can be especially hard to leave and to confront again the grief associated with letting go of primary care responsibilities.

Getting used to the new circumstances can be eased by making early visits relatively short, keeping conversations positive and staying with neutral topics that are not upsetting for the person with dementia. Communicating with body language that is relaxed and positive can help the person with dementia to be reassured that everything is OK. For residents with moderate or severe dementia, soft continuous recorded or live music, or gentle massage can be helpful to soothe and comfort them. Hymn singing or taking part in religious rituals can also help if that was part of the person's life before dementia. Some residents may enjoy a walk or other familiar activity that they usually find soothing. Leaving can be especially challenging if the person with dementia asks to go with you. The situation can be handled by reassuring and redirecting the person with dementia to another room or activity.

Many people feel uncomfortable about not being completely honest with someone with dementia. Is it OK to lie? In the 1990s a therapy called 'reality orientation' was popular in residential care. This therapy recommended bringing people with dementia 'back to reality', which sometimes upset people, especially if they were wondering where a deceased relative was and had to be told again that the person had passed away. The therapy has largely been replaced by 'validation therapy', which focuses instead on the underlying feelings behind agitated questioning (Feil 1993). So, for example, if someone with dementia is worried why someone is not visiting them, redirection and a gentle, 'He might be along later. Why don't we have a cup of tea now?' may be more calming than confronting the reality that the person is not coming right now.

When it is time to leave at the end of a visit, staff might assist you to disengage, perhaps by taking the person with dementia for a cup of tea or another activity to smooth your exit. Frequent one-to-one activities, where the resident has dedicated time with another family member, friend, staff member or volunteer doing something they enjoy, can be helpful. Knowing that the person with dementia will be engaged and relaxed after you leave can help to reassure family.

Even if your relative is confused and does not seem to make sense when you are visiting, listening to them and responding calmly can help them. Being with the person in a gentle and pleasant way is a good strategy at this time. How frequently you visit and how long you visit for will vary between families. For carers, you may want to visit your family member often, or you may need to share the visiting with other friends and family members who know your relative well, so that you can have time to recover from the process of being primary carer, which can often affect your own physical and mental health.

FOCUSING ON MEMORY ABILITIES RATHER THAN DISABILITIES

While dementia is a degenerative condition, some memory capacity remains, although it deteriorates over time. As a carer, it can help to remember to focus on the memories that are still there rather than the loss of memory. There is increasing recognition that memory can be supported and that not all memory is impaired in people with dementia. Some care homes may have psychologists available to assist with managing behaviours, such as repetitive questions and other symptoms that memory ability is deteriorating. For example, spaced retrieval is a psychological technique that has been used successfully with some people with dementia, to help them to remember important information by learning a procedure associated with the information (Oren, Willerton and Small 2014). A psychologist can help the person with dementia to learn important facts such as where the person lives now by learning to look at a diary whenever the person wishes to know the answer. The psychologist may start with one or two pieces of information to see whether the person with dementia is able to retain the information. Then the psychologist will have the person repeatedly practise giving a verbal response to the question and performing the activity of pulling their diary out of their pocket and reading it.

The technique uses a type of memory called procedural memory, which is unconscious and automatic. After successful spaced retrieval training, the person with dementia is able to unconsciously and automatically reach for the diary in their pocket to read the answer to the question. Memory is a complex part of brain function, and it is important to acknowledge that while memory functioning is impaired and deteriorating in someone living with dementia, there are parts of memory that will remain intact, and parts that can be supported to enable the person to function as well as possible. Some remarkable results have been found in using music to tap into memories of people with dementia, for example, and these activities can help to acknowledge the abilities that remain rather than the disabilities associated with dementia.

EASING THE TRANSITION FOR SOMEONE WITH DEMENTIA

Research has shown that the stress of moving into residential care can be eased by raising the subject early before the person with dementia has deteriorated, so the idea is less distressful for everyone. Planning practical strategies in advance and acknowledging the emotional impact of the change for everyone concerned can help them start to address ways to lessen the impact. Counselling for the family carer to help with the grief issues and to learn new ways of thinking about the situation can help. Starting to develop a relationship with staff that you trust in the care home will help to learn what the new partnership in care is going to be like and how you can continue to care without the added stress of day-to-day physical care. For the person with dementia, having their routines disturbed as little as possible, being surrounded by some familiar objects and photos, and having reassuring communication from staff will all help to adjust to the new situation. The family doctor also needs to be informed, and any medication decisions handed over to the next medical practitioner.

WHAT IS IT LIKE LIVING IN A HOME WITH PEOPLE WITH DEMENTIA?

For older people who do not have dementia, moving into a communal care setting such as a care home where many of the residents have memory loss can be confronting, and even frightening. When people move into residential care, the attitudes commonly found among the general public about dementia and Alzheimer's disease can easily have coloured their perception of the other residents. A number of public campaigns have targeted awareness about dementia and understanding, to reduce the stigma associated with the condition. Reports in both the UK and the USA have indicated that Alzheimer's disease and dementia are among the most feared diseases associated with getting older (Alzheimer's Disease International 2012). Stigma associated with dementia may even be higher among older people than among younger people (Cheston, Hancock and White 2016). Studies have shown that people have different attitudes to dementia depending on whether they have known someone with dementia before, and attitudes generally are reflected in the way people behave towards others (Cheston *et al.* 2016).

Interestingly, younger people may have more positive attitudes to dementia than older people. A study in Bristol and Gloucestershire showed that among 2201 people surveyed, younger men had more positive attitudes about dementia than either older men or older women. Many older people fear dementia, and some studies have shown that fear of dementia is greater than fear of cancer (Alzheimer's Disease International 2012). In some cultures, dementia is considered a mental illness and something shameful or to be hidden. Some people may feel that the odd behaviours associated with dementia are behaviours done 'on purpose' to threaten or intimidate others. Given the cultural and community fears associated with dementia, it is understandable that the prospect of living with people with dementia is very daunting for some people.

Despite common fears, living with someone who has dementia is not likely to cause an older person any harm. Many people with dementia are just the same as people who are more alert, and their disabilities in memory and thinking can sometimes be well hidden in social situations. Dementia is not contagious. It is important to see the person rather than the disease. People with early stage dementia may forget your name, but will be able to have a conversation and interact easily. In the middle stages, there may be some unusual behaviours occurring such as agitation and incontinence as the individual has lost ability to care for themselves. They may look dishevelled as the act of dressing becomes confusing for them, or they may remove some clothing in confusion about what time of day it is or where they are. They may enter your room thinking that it is their own. In fact, people with dementia are not acting in the way they do 'on purpose'.

How do you respond to these situations? Deliberately choosing your communication styles, it is important to respond calmly and in a friendly tone of voice, redirecting the person to their own room. While it can be annoying to have someone interfere with your routine or your things, it is not likely to be life threatening. Using your resilience skills, try not to consider the situation a catastrophe. Think of a goal that can help you to handle the situation, such as making an appointment to speak to the care manager about how they can support you in keeping a resident with dementia out of your room if it starts to happen frequently. Trying to remember your sense of humour can defuse a tense situation. Give yourself some praise for handling this unusual situation in a compassionate and calm way.

IAN AND PAT'S STORY

Ian and Pat's story illustrates that after admission to a care home, especially if you have been a carer yourself, it might be difficult to recognise that you also need to look after yourself, and that others can help you. If you move into care with your partner, it may take some time to deal with your own feelings associated with the move and other life changes. Remember that help is available to support you through this process.

Ian and Pat met as teenagers. They eventually married and raised a family. Ian described him and Pat as a team: he went out to paid work and Pat stayed at home and cared for their large family, and they also shared household chores. Sadly, Pat was diagnosed with dementia several years ago and her health has declined. Ian cared for Pat at home until he could no longer manage on his own, and felt that residential care was the best option: 'I said if we're going into a care home, I'm ready for that [too], I'll go with her.' After a time searching for a suitable place, Ian moved with Pat to a care home. Ian recalls thinking, 'I wouldn't care if I came here in the morning,' after the first time he visited the home he eventually moved to. 'I was impressed...the staff, the staff do impress me,' he adds.

At first, Ian found it very difficult to let the staff attend to Pat's care, explaining, '[It was] my job...I thought it was my duty to help her.' Ian felt a sense of disloyalty about allowing the staff to provide personal care to his wife, and resisted what he now recognises as the staff's kindness towards Pat, and to himself.

He explains it was a process of 'letting go' and handing over the care. The couple had spent over a year in the home before he felt he could let himself accept help and trust the staff to care for his wife. 'I finally did say there you are then, take care of her like I have all of these years.' He reflects, 'I was sort of protecting her, you know.' At the time of admission, and for many months afterwards, Ian was also experiencing intense feelings, including of anger and frustration at the situation the couple found themselves in due to dementia. 'Everything we did together...this disease has wrecked it; a good marriage and a friendship... Mentally, I was really, really, really [pauses]; that anger, I could have busted that door down... I cried buckets [of tears].' He also blames the disease for a loss of contact from friends and diminished family contact, although he feels supported at the care home, adding, 'This is my family now.'

Ian's health is now less robust, but he is comfortable with the living situation he and his wife have. He did not anticipate living in care until his wife became ill, but now he sees it as a supportive arrangement that works well for them both. 'I can walk into a home, and I can tell you there is love at home, yes,' he pauses, 'I can tell if there is love in the house. You get that feeling when you walk into a house, you know. I felt [it] here.'

Ian is a private person and is content to spend a bit of time on his own. When he was living at home, he did not have time to socialise, or enjoy his various interests. He now enjoys socialising with some of the other residents, and he feels there is plenty to do when he feels like it, including regular 'walks' outside with his wife. He enjoys doing things for himself when he can. 'Don't make yourself an invalid, don't say, "I can't",' is a philosophy he follows. Ian has found understanding support from the staff at the home, including the pastoral care practitioner, who visits him regularly, and with whom he feels he can really talk about how he is feeling. Ian is also writing his memoirs with the encouragement of the pastoral care practitioner, and he also now enjoys his long-neglected interests.

CHAPTER 8

DIVERSE NEEDS

For older people from diverse backgrounds it may be challenging to find care that suits their needs, so it is worth reflecting on what you feel your most important needs are, and to know your rights to having those needs respected. 'Diverse needs' is a term that recognises that everyone is unique and that there are individual differences that are important to take into account if we are to live life well. Our diverse needs can be due to race, ethnicity, gender, sexual orientation, religious or cultural beliefs, or other factors. Western societies are increasingly diverse, and this is reflected in the population of residents in care homes, as well as among the staff caring for them (Xiao *et al.* 2016). A recent census in Australia indicated that one in four Australians were born in another country (Australian Bureau of Statistics 2017). A broader recognition by western governments of the human rights of older people living in residential care means that there is now increased focus on how to meet the individual needs of people moving to residential care.

We all have unique care needs that relate to who we are and how we have lived our life, and with whom. The transition to residential care can be made more comfortable if an individual and their significant family members have their needs recognised and accommodated as far as is possible. Practically, this means with as little disruption to who you are and how you like to live as possible. Residential care providers cannot recognise your unique needs, though, unless you are aware of them yourself. This chapter will help you to reflect on what your unique needs are, and what the care home will need to recognise if they are to provide person-centred care for you (Yeboah 2015).

When you move to a care home, your life and the way you like to do things may become less private and seem more open to scrutiny. While living independently, your choice of lifestyle is something that you have developed over a long time. You may be wondering how well a care home is able to accommodate the way you like to live your life.

Moving to a care home gives you an opportunity to reflect on what is most important to you, and what defines your identity as 'you'. You may have concerns about being able to do the things you like to do, and also concerns that there are some things that you will no longer be able to do at all. This chapter will focus on some common areas of 'diversity' that may impact on moving into residential care: sexuality, religion and spirituality, culture, ethnic diversity, gender and veterans. Men's rights as residents of residential care are discussed, as men tend to be a minority group in care homes, compared with women. These areas of diversity in residential care do not make up an exhaustive list. It is intended that discussion of these common areas of diversity will help you think about your own diverse needs and about how to get the best care to suit those needs.

WHAT IS 'PERSON-CENTRED CARE'?

One of the main concerns for people moving to residential care is whether they will get the sort of care they need, in the way they want it. This essentially describes what 'person-centred care' is; it requires a focus by service providers on an individual, their way of life, and supporting their independence and the way they like to live their life (Dow *et al.* 2006). Person-centred care is achieved by care home providers making a genuine attempt to meet the needs and preferences of that person. It recognises that the person who has moved to residential care is not only an individual, but also someone who has been a part of a family, social group or community, who wishes to remain so as much as possible, in an environment that is as familiar as possible (Dow *et al.* 2006). Well-trained staff recognise that how a person chooses to be 'independent' and 'autonomous' will depend on their personal experience and cultural perspective. For example, some people like their families to make decisions for them, and to advocate for them. If this is how you or your family member moving to care likes to make decisions and be supported by family, it is important to tell staff that this is what you want, and ensure they appreciate its significance to you. Talking with your family doctor and senior care staff may help junior staff to appreciate your need more fully.

The right to participate in your own health and social care includes your right to indicate how you would like health and social care decisions concerning you to be made, as well as your right to participate in decisions about what care you may want.

Ask the care home to explain your rights regarding:
- decisions about your care, both on a day-to-day basis and more formally
- expression of culture, religion, sexuality and other diverse needs.

Some residential care homes meet the needs of their residents better than other care homes. This can be for a variety of reasons, including the underlying organisational values influencing the care home, the way government policy and care standards have been interpreted and implemented at the care home, and management practices. The level of training and support of staff, and staff skills and care delivery also influence the care provided to people moving into care homes.

HUMAN RIGHTS AND CARE HOME RESIDENTS

Human rights are rights that everyone is entitled to regardless of their age, citizenship, nationality, race, ethnicity, gender, sexuality, religion, language, abilities or any other status (HelpAge International 2010a, 2010b). The Universal Declaration of Human Rights has existed since 1948 and has now become recognised as law that is binding in all countries. The UK became a signatory to the European Convention of Human Rights in 1951, but it is only recently that human rights law has been considered specifically in relation to the human rights of older people in a care home context, and in the wider community (Doyle and Roberts 2016a). Your care home will have a statement of your rights and you and your family should familiarise yourself with them.

Increasingly, older people and their families are comfortable with becoming more assertive and raising their expectations of their residential care experience, and their political clout has also become more recognised by governments. Human rights for older people in a care context mean that they can expect particular care experiences, including a right to self-expression. This includes the right to engage in decision making about their care as much as is possible, to refuse care they do not want (within the existing law) and to express the care that they may want that accords with their values. Older people, including those living in care homes, may require special care and support to ensure that they are protected from elder abuse, which may be financial, but may also be emotional and physical, in the form of 'cruel, inhuman or degrading treatment or punishment' (United Nations General Assembly 1987).

Know your rights when moving into a care home, as this will help you know what is reasonable to expect and what is unreasonable to expect. In Australia, the Office of the Public Advocate in Victoria can provide more information about your rights in that state, and My Aged Care is the Australian government body that can provide a lot of information about care and your rights. In the UK, Age UK has information about your rights. Health professionals such as social workers, community workers, local council care officers, family doctors, community care nurses and care assessment teams should also be able to discuss your rights.

CULTURAL AND LINGUISTIC DIVERSITY

'Culture' is everything that makes and shapes you and influences who you are: your ethnicity, your language, your social customs and behaviours, your beliefs and your religion, if you have a particular religious faith. It might also mean your spirituality, or 'source of meaning' that drives you and gives you purpose in life. How important is your cultural background in your life? We encourage you to consider these important aspects of who you are when moving to a care home. Some people will choose to live in an ethno-specific care home, for example, a care home for Chinese residents, or for Italian or Greek residents. Others may choose to live in a religion-specific care home, for example, a home for Catholic or Jewish residents. Such choices will be a reflection of priority for the residents who choose these. If culture or language choices are important to you or your family, then ask how they can be maintained in the care home. If family gatherings are part of your life, then check with the care home how they can include families (including larger families) who want to visit and to be involved in the day-to-day activities of the care home, as this can give an indication of the openness and flexibility of a care home to accommodate residents' needs. This is an indicator of true 'person-centred care'.

Another important aspect of having your diverse needs met regarding culture in a care home is getting the food you like. Explore what sort of food is provided at the care homes you are considering a move to. Ask what the policy is regarding residents' family members bringing in food, too. Check whether you are able to order in the type of food you like, when you like, if the food you prefer is not routinely offered at the care home. It is a fair question to ask care home senior management why they cannot be more culturally responsive to the diverse food preferences of their residents.

Find out if the care home celebrates multicultural events, and whether the cultural days and events important to you – for example, Christmas, Passover or Diwali – are celebrated at the care home or somewhere close by that you can attend if you wish. It is also helpful to check if there is a pastoral care practitioner who either works at the care home, or who visits regularly, as they are trained to support you in the way you wish to live your life by helping to honour what is important to you, be it observing a religion or some other important spiritual practice.

For people who have little family support, it is especially important to have access to pastoral care. It might come from a visiting religious leader or a special health worker or another health professional with special training.

If you have been unwell, you may rely on others to help you do this searching regarding getting your cultural needs met. Speak to people who know you best and who know what is important to you.

SPIRITUALITY AND RELIGION

Beyond seeking a care home that caters specifically to your religion, what else is important in acknowledging your diverse needs regarding spirituality? This might be a challenging question to ask yourself, and to reflect on.

Spirituality can be an uncomfortable term for people to think about and to discuss with others. It is challenging for people living in care when staff associate spirituality with religion only. For many people, spiritual care is not necessarily just religious care. All care homes should provide some pastoral care that addresses the individual's spiritual needs through the way staff respond to residents, the way diverse needs are catered for, the way meaning and hope are provided and the way connectedness with others is given attention. Australia recently adopted some guidelines for spiritual care in residential care which list some outcomes and actions that care providers can use to assess whether their care is paying enough attention to the spiritual needs of their residents (Meaningful Ageing Australia 2016).

KULWANT'S STORY

Kulwant's story illustrates that grief is difficult for everyone, and especially for people of cultural and linguistic diversity who may feel misunderstood and socially isolated, as can be the case when one moves to a care home. When the person moving into care has not had much or any control over the decision to move, does not confidently speak English as a first language, and where the care staff and many residents are not of the same cultural background, expect an added layer of grief that will require gentle care while the person transitions to their new place of residence. Anything that connects the person to their own culture (including language) will provide some comfort, as will the ability for the person who has moved to be with and talk with someone of their own cultural background or someone who is a close friend. Families will also need support for their grief.

Kulwant, the matriarch of a large Sikh family living in metropolitan Sydney, Australia, was very reluctantly moved to a residential care home directly from respite care when her elderly husband, Raj, who was her main carer, died suddenly. Kulwant and her husband had moved from India to be with their family 15 years ago. Kulwant's family were close and caring, but even so, they were unable to be with Kulwant all day due to work and other family commitments. The family felt very guilty about this and felt they had failed their mother by moving her to a care home. Kulwant had always been quite independent, but her vascular dementia had steadily become worse, especially since the death of her husband, for whom she (and her family) were deeply grieving. She had managed activities at home, such as walking around the garden, reading the newspaper, eating and showering, but she relied almost completely on others for planning home management and activities such as bill paying, cleaning and cooking.

Once in care, Kulwant wandered around and wanted to 'go home' to her (recently deceased) husband. She did not understand why no one would help her do so. This distressed her – and her family. The care home manager, Elizabeth, encouraged Kulwant's family to take her on a visit to her family home in Sydney, and to take her to the local Sikh temple to visit friends and to pray, as she had done for many years on a regular basis. She also listened to and encouraged the family's ideas about how Kulwant could best be kept as connected as possible with the Sikh community and her neighbours, with whom she had close bonds. She helped Kulwant keep participating in the hobbies she had enjoyed, such as reading, and watching funny Hindi movies. Kulwant noticed a Punjabi lady working in the care home and they started conversing on a regular basis in the Punjabi language, which they both seemed to enjoy. Kulwant's family brought her favourite food to her whenever they visited and were also able to arrange for regular delivery of Punjabi food to Kulwant, from a local caterer and the care home kitchen staff. The family was also able to put family photos on Kulwant's walls, as well as familiar decorations, so she felt more, 'at home'. They brought her in her favourite music and favourite chair, too.

Over time, many of the residents enjoyed the semi-regular 'curry nights', which were part of the care home's activities to embrace multiculturalism, along with Italian, Greek and other cuisine 'nights'. The staff and Kulwant's family encouraged Kulwant to keep watching her beloved football team on TV, and staff introduced her to another woman in the care home who followed the same team. They started watching football and cricket together and seemed to enjoy each other's company while doing this. Over time, Kulwant, who was now receiving regular visits from friends, became less agitated, and did not ask as often if she could 'go home', although she did go on occasional drives with her family to familiar parts of Sydney, at which time she reminisced and sometimes cried, as she missed her husband very much. A few months later, just before the time of Diwali celebrations, Elizabeth's staff asked Kulwant's family how best they might help Kulwant and her fellow care home residents celebrate this occasion. Kulwant's family were delighted by this request, and quick to give advice and practical assistance, as was Kulwant.

SEXUALITY AND GENDER

The prospect of communal living may be especially confronting when considering issues of sexuality and gender. The term 'sexuality' will mean different things to different people. Here, we are referring to a person's sexual orientation and preferred expression of that orientation, as well as the way they wish to express the sexual aspect of their 'being' or 'humanness'. Sexual expression can be encompassed by terms such as heterosexual, same-sex attracted (lesbian and gay), bisexual and more. Some people may not identify with any particular term or description, but nevertheless consider themselves 'sexual beings'. Gender should also be taken into account, whether the person is cisgender, transgender, non-binary, gender-queer or identifies in another way.

We recognise now that there are many ways that a person can experience and express their sexuality. Some would argue that they no longer wish to think about sexuality in later life, while others consider that it continues to be an essential part of who they are and the more overtly they are able to express their sexuality, the better. Then there are all the other people in between on a very long continuum, and their preferences for means of sexual expression may change at times. Some people entering residential care might consider the intimacy of close discussion, an intellectual 'connection' with another, a verbal flirtation or being quietly in the presence of another they are attracted to as 'expressing their sexuality'. Other people may require their sexuality to be much more openly expressed, and may need to be more physically demonstrative of affection and intimacy with a partner. For some people, including those who have not had a partner, or cannot see their partner as often as they wish, their sexuality may also be expressed alone in a private space.

As a general principle, unfortunately residential care is not as accommodating or supportive of residents' sexual expression as it could be, or, many would say, should be (Mahieu and Gastmans 2015; Bauer *et al.* 2007, 2014). There are exceptions and, in policy terms, things are improving to support residents in care to be able to express themselves as they wish. Part of this change is through a recognition of older people's human rights.

Staff training and attitudes will have considerable bearing on how well they support residents to express themselves sexually (Mahieu and Gastmans 2015; Villar *et al.* 2015). If you have concerns that a care home may not support your needs for sexual expression, it is worth asking some questions and doing some 'detective work' for yourself or your family member moving into care. This can be difficult to talk about with family and care home staff, but if it is important to you, then you need to be bold if you possibly can be, as some care homes unfortunately still treat residents as if they are 'sexuality-less' beings with no need for privacy, let alone sexual expression. For some family members, this may be a 'no go' zone from a conversational point of view, but other families and family members will be more willing to broach the subject with their family member going into residential care, and with the senior staff at the care home. An assertive friend who is willing to support you can be invaluable in these circumstances, as can be a sensitive social worker, pastoral care practitioner or family doctor. Lesbian, gay, bisexual, transgender, intersex and questioning (LGBTIQ) support agencies may also have workers who can help identify more LGBTIQ-sensitive care homes.

Some basic questions might include: how much privacy residents are given if they want to meet with a partner who is also a resident, or who visits periodically, to behave in an 'adult' fashion. Are there locks on the door of the residents' rooms? Is there a protocol for not disturbing residents if they wish to have private time either alone or with a partner?

For people who identify as LGBTIQ, you may also wish to ask if there is a policy for the care and support of people who identify as LGBTIQ, and whether there are other people in the care home who are LGBTIQ. If the answer is a bewildered or embarrassed response, a 'no' or an 'I don't know', this can be a warning signal that the care home does not have LGBTIQ-identifying people on its radar, and an LGBTIQ person moving to that home may feel that the sexual side of their being will be ignored or actively denied expression by the care home staff.

Another important area for LGBTIQ-identifying people living in care is recognition of their same-sex or LGBTIQ partner as their 'partner'. It can be very hurtful if their partner is not acknowledged as such when they want them to be, especially when the lack of recognition would be far less likely to happen if the care home resident were in a heterosexual relationship. This can be especially important when an LGBTIQ-identifying person expects that their partner will be their formal health care decision maker if and when they lack the cognitive ability to make their own health care decisions, in the context of broader family denial of the relationship the person living in care has with their LGBTIQ partner. See Chapter 3 for more information about this.

NORMAN'S STORY

Norman's story illustrates that staff are interested in supporting you to meet your need for particular care. Some staff are not as sensitive or as well trained as others. Sometimes, it can be as simple as being able to ask staff about something that you find a bit difficult to talk about. At other times, you may feel that staff are not interested in hearing you, or you may not know how to raise a subject, such as your needs for physical intimacy or privacy. If you are finding it difficult to have a conversation with any of the staff about a particular need you have, talk to a trusted family member, friend, family doctor, other health care professional or pastoral care practitioner and arrange to get some support from them or someone else who can advocate for you. You do have the right to ask to have your needs met, and some care home management staff might need a nudge to respond to the unrecognised needs of their residents.

Norman, an inquisitive and gentle man, lived independently for many years with his wife, Meg. Meg was visually impaired and her worsening osteoarthritis was increasingly limiting her ability to walk very far, or to use her hands. After debilitating back problems necessitating spinal surgery, Norman became wheelchair-bound and was no longer able to stay living at home due to this and other health problems. He moved into residential care, and his wife moved into their daughter's home. This physical separation was distressing for both Norman and Meg, but they were determined to 'make the best of it'. In some areas, Norman and Meg may have had the option of moving into a care home together, perhaps with a shared unit or adjoining rooms. For Norman and Meg, this was not an option.

Norman missed his wife, and shared with his visiting agency nurse that he missed the physical side of the relationship with his wife. He told the nurse he craved that intimacy, and felt as if they did not have any opportunity for privacy when his wife visited him. He explained that there were no locks on the door, staff often interrupted them and that the staff never raised the issue of providing privacy to him, or to him and his wife during their time together. He was not sure that he could ask, but he did ask his visiting agency nurse whether it would be 'wrong' if he used 'phone sex' services to help him with his feelings of sexual frustration. He explained that he had thought about it, but did not want to be 'disloyal' to his beloved wife. His agency nurse offered to tactfully raise the issue of providing a safe and private environment for Norman and Meg during Meg's visits, and whenever Norman required privacy, and he was encouraged by the nurse to express his needs to a sensitive staff member, who then became aware that he had unmet needs. The care home eventually provided training for all staff around the needs for privacy, sexual expression and intimacy for all residents. Some staff were uncomfortable about this training, but were supported to understand why it was important for the residents' health and well-being.

BEING IN THE MINORITY: MEN IN CARE HOMES

In residential care, men are a minority group compared with women. Some men living in care can feel that there are limited opportunities for them to meet and socialise with other men. Care home staff are mainly women too. So, if you are a man who has just moved to a care home, finding out who the other men there are, both residents and staff, can make you feel more comfortable in your new surroundings and will help you find out what activities and social opportunities there are to socialise with other men, as well as women, at the care home, based on your interests.

Some care homes have regular 'men only' activity groups and social occasions such as watching sport together or playing cards, snooker or boules. In Australia, some residential care homes have 'men's sheds' or 'man caves', where groups of men can meet and participate in activities such as woodwork or repairs, or make things in the way they did when they were living at home and had their own 'shed'. Such activities can provide purpose, meaning and connection with others. Men's activities are often initiated by thoughtful staff, or developed by residents with the assistance of staff, or it might be a collaborative effort. Family can help with instigating such activities, too, if they get to know the staff and the resident requires an advocate to help engage them with their new surroundings and care community.

Some men decide to move to residential care if their partner requires care. Men in these circumstances may have been the carer of their partner and their own health may also have deteriorated. They may be feeling exhausted, guilty and in need of emotional support, even if they do not realise it immediately. For some men (and women), it is difficult to even realise what needs they have if they have been 'caring' for someone else for a while.

Men living in a care home, either with their partner or alone, may be less likely to express their needs if it is not something they have ever done. It can seem difficult to say how you are feeling to relative strangers; however, it can be a most liberating thing if you find a compassionate and caring staff member, such as a pastoral care worker or other suitably trained and experienced staff. Talking with trained and experienced staff members can reduce the sense of isolation and loneliness that can cause a range of difficult feelings when you move to residential care, with or without your partner.

SPECIAL NEEDS OF VETERANS

Most veterans are likely to reside in a care home that has many non-veterans living in it too. For some veterans, it may not seem as important as for others to identify as 'a veteran'. It will depend on the veteran and their personal experience. To ensure that the care home you choose will meet *your* needs as a veteran, it might be helpful to ask the care home how many, or what percentage of their existing residents are veterans, and how much experience the care home has with caring for veterans. It is also worth asking how the care home supports its veteran population and whether they have a policy around caring for veterans. For example, are they strongly linked with external services available to veterans? Blank looks from the staff when you ask such questions may indicate that they do not understand the special needs veteran have, or that a significant move like that to a care home might trigger some unpleasant memories associated with grief and past trauma. Access to the company of other veterans, as well as access to adequate mental health services and quiet spaces, may be especially helpful. So, too, might the recognition and appropriate honouring of significant days such as ANZAC day in Australia and Remembrance Sunday in the UK, and other dates worldwide that are etched in the memories of veterans and their families.

Some veterans may have post-traumatic stress disorder (PTSD), and in older generations of veterans, PTSD is poorly recognised and diagnosed. PTSD can be associated with reliving the traumatic event often in the form of nightmares, or physical reactions such as sweating, heart palpitations or panic when reminded of the event. Some people with PTSD experience sleep difficulties, irritability and lack of concentration, and are easily startled. Sometimes people deliberately avoid being reminded of the event because it brings back painful memories. People may feel emotionally numb and cut off from friends or family, and lose interest in daily activities.

For some veterans moving to residential care, it can be uncomfortable or 'triggering' to have care staff of particular nationalities caring for them, if they have fought against people of those nationalities in the past. This is not always the case for every veteran, but if this does occur, staff should be sympathetic and understanding of past trauma experienced by veterans. For veterans who have cognitive impairment, perhaps due to dementia, this behaviour might be more evident, but it will, of course, depend on the individual resident and their experience. It is worth talking with the staff of a care home you or your family member are considering moving to, to check how they have handled such circumstances. Importantly, female and male veterans may have differing needs, and it may be that female veterans might wish to socialise with other female veterans, if this is possible. Generally, sensitive and well-trained staff who are guided by thoughtful policy will be able to meet the needs of veterans living in care, if they have access to suitable support services.

CHAPTER 9

COPING WITH DEATH AND DYING IN CARE HOMES

Many people are fearful of moving into residential care because they fear they are going there to die. The colloquial phrase 'God's waiting room' is sometimes used in a derogatory way to refer to care homes as places where nothing is happening and people who are living there are simply waiting to die – a truly grim prospect. This negative view of care homes colours our perceptions and feeds into fear of what to expect and how to handle our new identity associated with living in a care home. In fact, most people who move into residential care do die there. In Australia, most permanent residents (91 per cent) leave the home at death. A small proportion (4 per cent) move back to the community; about half of those people who move back to the community have only lived in residential care for less than three months (Australian Institute of Health and Welfare 2012).

The remainder of residents leave to go to hospital and do not return, dying in hospital, or they go to an alternative care home. The life of older people living in a care home before death can be made as pleasant an experience as possible by attending to the strategies discussed in this book. But death is inevitable, and dying in the hands of experts, people who know you and loved ones is probably preferable to the uncertain experience of death elsewhere. If you have an advance care plan, you are more likely to be cared for and to die in the way that you had wished to. In a care home, staff can strive to help the individual to have a 'good death', as comfortable an experience as possible for themselves, their families and the people around them, other residents and staff. In this chapter, we discuss how residential care homes provide support to enable end-of-life care to be as good as possible.

END-OF-LIFE CARE PATHWAY

In deciding about care in advance (see Chapter 3), some residents will elect to be moved to an 'end-of-life care pathway' when they are dying. This is a term for palliative care and a planned approach to end-of-life care. Palliative care is care that ensures maximum comfort to a person. It is provided when people have an advanced terminal illness at the end of life, and also to some people with a serious chronic illness that is unlikely to be cured even before they are actively dying. The approach aims to keep the quality of life as good as possible, through medical and nursing care, and neither shorten nor extend life through treatments that are offered. It can occur over many months or just for a short time. Staff at the care home will discuss all care options with the individual and their substitute decision maker or 'person responsible'.

An end-of-life care pathway will be initiated by staff in consultation with the individual, their family and their medical practitioner. In many cases the pathway will enable the person to remain in the care home rather than be transferred to hospital, if that is their wish. Some people may prefer to be transferred to hospital and to have every effort made to extend their life using all available technology, but this is not the choice everyone will make and hospitals are not obliged to provide care that is deemed 'futile', although this can be a controversial point for some. Deciding on this in advance is part of the advance care plan process. The pathway will also pay special attention to the spiritual and psychological preferences of the individual. At the end of life, the physical and social environment can be especially important in providing comfort to the individual, their family and friends. Apart from medical and nursing considerations, details such as the presence or absence of music, pastoral care practitioners, special ceremonial artefacts and even pets can be specified in advance to help the individual to maintain control over the last stage of their life.

Not everyone has experienced a death of someone close to them. The care home may have a brochure for relatives and friends to help them to understand the dying process, although brochures may not be the best way for everyone to learn about this sensitive subject. Many younger relatives may not have experienced someone dying before, and knowing some of what to expect can help them to cope with the experience. Older people themselves have often had more experience with friends dying, and have a more accepting, less anxious view of death than their younger relatives. For some older people who are anxious about death, knowing what might be expected and feeling as though they have some control over what will happen will be comforting.

SAYING GOODBYE TO OTHER RESIDENTS

It is highly likely that other residents will die during your stay in residential care. It can be hard to say goodbye to residents who have become friends, and difficult to see a favourite chair vacant or to find that a room that was always known as one person's haven, their home, is now occupied by a new face. These daily realities of living in a care home can be glossed over by some staff, especially those who have difficulty facing the loss of a resident themselves. Some staff may feel uncomfortable to see older residents expressing emotion through crying and may shy away from talking about someone's death for fear of upsetting residents. It may be that the residents teach staff how to openly express acceptance of death, and that death is not to be feared or hidden. Many care staff admire the wisdom and experience of their residents.

Some care homes have processes in place to honour the passing of a resident, and ceremonies and memorials can be a comforting way to mark the death of a resident, regardless of whether those concerned had a particular religious faith or spiritual background. Being able to celebrate the life of a friend, to remember their good qualities and the fun times that were had with the individual can help everyone in the community to say goodbye and accept the death as part of the cycle of life. It can also be comforting to people left behind in the home, knowing that when their turn comes they will also be remembered in a similar way, and not be immediately forgotten or ignored after the last stage of their life.

UNDERSTANDING GRIEF

There are many losses experienced throughout life, each of them unique, and for people moving into residential care and for their families, understanding grief and loss can be particularly relevant to their experience and stage of life.

How each loss is experienced and adjusted to will also be unique. Even as we age, losses associated with moving house, loss of independence, even loss of ability to carry out tasks independently and loss of independence in bodily functions all require some adjustment and working out how to continue living without what we had before. Losing a friend in residential care or a family member is another significant loss to be adjusted to, and grief is experienced differently by everyone. It can be overwhelming, and feel never-ending, but it is important to understand our own reactions and to find ways to allow ourselves to recover.

There is no right or wrong way to grieve, and no prescription on how long grief will last or how long someone should take to recover from a loss. Grief will affect feelings, thoughts, physical symptoms, relationships, behaviours and beliefs (Palliative Care Australia 2017). Feelings such as shock, sadness, anger and anxiety are common. Some people have difficulty concentrating, and thoughts about the person who passed away may intrude on everyday tasks, and even during sleep, with dreams about the person being experienced. Stress associated with grief can often be experienced as tiredness, and other physical symptoms such as nausea, loss of appetite or pain can be signs of grief, but they may also be signs of physical illness so they should be checked by a health practitioner. Relationships with other people can be affected by the grieving process, as someone who is grieving may be disengaged from others or seem distracted or uninterested. Some people who are grieving may find it hard to look after themselves and seek to dampen strong feelings with alcohol or painkillers. Some people find that their religious belief framework is challenged by grief, as they struggle to understand why a person has been taken from them. People can feel isolated and lonely in their grief, so sharing the above reactions with someone can help to ease the feeling that grieving is a lonely journey.

Elizabeth Kubler-Ross (2005) identified five stages of grief: denial (this can't be happening); anger (why is this happening?); bargaining (make this not happen and in return I will...); depression (I'm too sad to do anything); and acceptance (I'm at peace with what happened). Many people experience some of these stages, and while they may not happen in a straight line and were not intended to describe a 'normal' response, over time most people will come to accept their loss.

WAYS TO HELP WITH COPING WITH GRIEF

There are many tips that have been suggested as ways to help with coping with grief (HelpGuide 2017).

It can help to acknowledge that you have experienced a loss, and seek some support from the people who care about you – talk to them or just be with them. If you don't have anyone close in the care home, then now is the time to reach out to a staff member or a volunteer to help you with your response to grief. If there is no one you would feel comfortable talking to, then joining a counselling or support group can help you share with others who have experienced a loss. In the care home setting this group may be reminiscing about the person who died, and sharing your feelings with the group or just hearing how others have responded to the loss can assist with processing your own feelings. If groups do not suit you as an individual, then talk to a therapist, grief counsellor or pastoral care practitioner – someone who is an experienced counsellor can help you to work through the experience.

Some people find comfort in faith – rituals, ceremonies and spiritual activities can help some people in their grief – and some care homes offer special masses or ceremonies to celebrate the life of the person who died.

At a personal level, mindfulness or noticing and accepting that you are feeling emotions can help to resolve them over time. Writing feelings down in a journal or writing a letter can help to express how the loss has affected you. At the same time, it is important to look after your physical health – if you are experiencing physical symptoms, see a medical practitioner or speak to the care staff who can help to monitor the impact of grief on your own health. Finally, at times of grief it can help to try to maintain a routine – hobbies, routines and 'putting one foot in front of the other' can help to get through the day.

Some other suggestions from Palliative Care Australia (2017) include talking to the person who has died (to yourself), looking at photos or visiting special places that you shared with them to keep the memories alive. Sometimes reading about other people's experiences of grief and how they handled it can help to understand the process you are going through, and meditation or massage or other self-care experiences may be helpful to look after yourself during this difficult time.

Things that may *not* help someone who is grieving:
- stopping contact with the person who is grieving is not usually helpful
- being offended by their changed or angry mood, which can be a way of expressing pain and grief
- telling the person you know how they feel is not accurate – everyone is different
- giving them advice about how they should be acting may be taken as a criticism
- avoiding their grief by being jolly or trying to cheer someone up is not usually helpful
- avoiding mentioning the person who died (unless that is culturally appropriate)
- trying to look on the bright side.

Adapted from Palliative Care Australia (2017)

THE DIFFERENCE BETWEEN GRIEF AND DEPRESSION

Grief and depression can share some symptoms, but while grief can affect our emotions like a roller coaster, the symptoms of depression are more constant. It is important to check with a health professional if grief seems to be overlaid with depression. Symptoms of depression that are not normally considered part of grieving include: thoughts of suicide, feeling hopeless or worthless, slower speech or body movements and intense feelings of guilt. It is not normally recommended that anti-depressants are prescribed for grief, but it is important to speak to a mental health professional if symptoms of grief are distressing, to make sure that your own health is not affected.

If you are feeling suicidal seek help immediately. Call a suicide prevention helpline:

In the UK – 08457 90 90 90

In the USA – 1 800 273 TALK (8255)

In Canada – www.suicideprevention.ca/need-help

In Australia – 13 11 14

CHAPTER 10

SUMMING UP

The move to a residential care home can be a challenging and demanding transition on many levels both for the person moving and for their families and friends helping them. It requires significant renegotiation on the part of the new resident and their family members to adjust to the new living situation, and from a psychological point of view it may mean taking on a new identity while retaining all the parts of life that made up the essential 'you'. Most people will adjust to the change and, using some of the strategies recommended in this book, will come to accept that on balance it was the best option and that there are some aspects of the new life that are enjoyable. You may surprise yourself at how strong and resilient you have become as a result of adjusting to this major life event. Or you may have found out something new about yourself when you thought there was nothing new to be learned.

Some of the factors that can influence how a person responds to the transition to residential care include:

- whether or not the person decided for themselves that they needed support from a care home
- whether the person agrees to or understands that they need residential care

- whether the person requiring care is able to participate meaningfully in the decision making process about moving, and to what extent
- how much time the person and their family has to talk about and plan the move
- the personal resilience of the new resident
- the past experiences of change of the new resident
- the person's ability and willingness to foster new social relationships
- the person's ability to maintain existing relationships.

None of the above factors concerns the quality of care offered in the care home. The other group of factors affecting the transition experience involves the contribution of the care home and the staff, and how they handle the introduction of a new resident. These factors include:

- the fit between resident need and care home service provision
- the level of support they and their families receive
- the admission processes at the care home
- staff attitudes to caring
- the physical environment of the care home
- the other residents in the home; how well they match the new resident and how much they have in common with the new resident.

Then there are factors added to the equation by the resident's social support, family or friends:

- whether the new resident had any social support before they moved into the care home

- how accepting their family or friends are about the new situation
- their family's attitude to the care home and its practices and staff
- how well they handle the change in situation for their family member
- how past dynamics in the relationship with the older person impact on the way new issues are handled
- how stresses in their own lives impact on they way they handle the move.

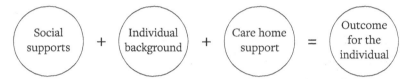

Figure 10.1: The outcome of adjusting to living in a care home depending on three groups of factors in the equation

Some people with no social support but great personal resilience will adapt to change no matter what. Others may have great social support and a good care home environment that can bolster them to produce a good outcome. The sum of these three groups of factors – social supports from family, individual background and care home approach to support – will combine to produce the outcome for the individual resident and how well they fare in their new environment.

Moving to a residential care home is a big challenge for many older people and their families. Challenges and situations that may never have been experienced before can test resilience and strength. At the same time, memorable experiences can be had, some new friendships can be forged and comforting memories made. Usually, most people adjust to their new home, and most have made the right choice for them. Some make new friends, many feel safe and well cared for, and many are satisfied that, despite the restrictions of disability or ill health, the move has enabled them to continue to live their life with some comfort and enjoyment, a common goal for all of us.

INTERNET AND TELEPHONE RESOURCES ABOUT MOVING INTO RESIDENTIAL CARE

UK

Action on Elder Abuse
https://elderabuse.org.uk – Confidential help and advice on all aspects of elder abuse. Tel: 080 8808 8141

Age UK
www.ageuk.org/home-and-care/care-homes/finding-a-care-home/#whattoask – A video and checklist of questions to ask when seeking a care home

www.ageuk.org.uk/no-one/we-provide-advice – Information and advice on a variety of topics related to aged care. Advice line – Tel: 0800 678 1174

Alzheimer's Society
www.alzheimers.org.uk/downloads/download/1125/factsheet_selecting_a_care_home – Factsheet on choosing a care home for someone with dementia

www.alzheimers.org.uk/info/20012/helpline – National dementia helpline for information, support or advice about dementia. Tel: 0300 222 11 22

Anchor

www.anchor.org.uk/help-and-guides/guide-to-choosing-a-care-home/care-home-selection-checklist – A not-for-profit provider with information about choosing a care home

Care UK

www.careuk.com/care-homes – A care provider with information about choosing care

Compassion in Dying UK

www.compassionindying.org.uk – Tel: 0800 999 2434. Information about making decisions and planning your care

HOPEline UK

Tel: 0800 0684141 – Practical advice on suicide prevention

Independent Age

www.independentage.org/information/support-care/care-homes/choosing-right-care-home – Information about choosing a case home and deciding on priorities

National Council for Palliative Care

www.ncpc.org.uk/publication/planning-your-future-care – Tel: 0207 6971520. 'Planning for your future care guide 2014'. Updated version explains advance care planning and providing information and resources about the advance care planning process

NHS Choices

www.nhs.uk/Conditions/social-care-and-support-guide/Pages/care-homes.aspx – Basic information about care homes and choices

www.nhs.uk/conditions/counselling/pages/introduction.aspx – Information on availability of carer counselling services

www.nhs.uk/Conditions/Suicide/Pages/Getting-help.aspc – Information about getting help if you are feeling suicidal
www.nhs.uk/Planners/end-of-life-care/Pages/planning-ahead. aspx – End-of-life care and advance care planning. Information on planning for your future care, including advance care planning and advance directives, and service locations

SupportLine
www.supportline.org.uk/problems/bereavement.php – Tel: 01708 765200. Support line for a range of problems related to bereavement and grief

Samaritans
Tel: 116 123 – 24-hour telephone counselling service

Which?
www.which.co.uk/elderly-care – Information and advice about care homes

USA AND CANADA

AARP (American Association of Retired Persons)
www.aarp.org/home-family/caregiving/info-2016/aarp-local-caregiver-resource-guides.html – Separate caregiver resource guides by state

www.aarp.org/home-family/caregiving/info-05-2012/caregiving-resource-center-asking-right-questions.html – A checklist for choosing a long-term care home in the USA

Aging Parents and Elder Care
www.aging-parents-and-elder-care.com/Pages/Checklists/
Alzheimers_Chklst.html – A checklist for choosing a dementia
facility or care home

www.aging-parents-and-elder-care.com/Pages/Checklists/
Nursing_Home.html – A nursing home checklist

Alzheimer's Association
www.alz.org/visitinganursinghome.pdf – Points on choosing a
nursing home in the USA

Alzheimer Society Canada
www.alzheimer.ca/en/Living-with-dementia/caring-for-
someone/long-term-care/finding-a-home – Points about finding
the right home

A Place for Mom
www.aplaceformom.com/search – Information about housing
options by state in USA and province in Canada

www.aplaceformom.com/senior-care-resources#checklist –
Checklists for finding nursing homes and other information

British Columbia government, Canada
www2.gov.bc.ca/gov/content/family-social-supports/seniors/
health-safety/advance-care-planning – Telephone HealthLink
BC, toll free at 8 1 1 (dial 7 1 1 for deaf and hearing-impaired
assistance). British Columbia government website about
advance care planning for people of cultural and linguistic
diversity

California Courts
www.courts.ca.gov/1058.htm – Self-help information for victims of abuse (California)

Elder Abuse NYC
http://nyceac.com – Support and information for people regarding elder abuse (New York City)

Elder Abuse Ontario
www.elderabuseontario.com – Telephone Seniors Safety Line toll free: 1 866 299 1011. Support and information line for seniors about elder abuse (Ontario, Canada)

Elder Law Answers
www.elderlawanswers.com/checklist-factors-to-consider-in-selecting-a-nursing-home-12146 – A checklist of factors to consider in selecting a nursing home

Medicare
www.medicare.gov/nursinghomecompare/search.html – A guide to choosing a nursing home or other long-term services and supports

National Domestic Violence Hotline (including elder abuse)
Tel: 1 800 799 7233; TDD: 1 800 787 3224 – Links people to resources and support in their community

National Hospice and Palliative Care Organization
www.caringinfo.org – Tel: 1 800 658 8898 (toll free); 1 877 658 8896 (toll free/multilingual). Free resources to help people make decisions about end-of-life care, including advance care planning

National Institute on Aging

www.nia.nih.gov/health/caregiving/advance-care-planning –
Comprehensive information and resources about advance care
planning, and contact details in various states

Ontario government, Canada

www.ontario.ca/page/health-and-wellness-information-seniors –
Tel: 1 888 910 1999; TTY/Teletypewriter: 1 800 387 5559. Seniors
Affairs, Ontario government information website for seniors,
covering a range of topics including advance care planning and
dementia

Seniors Abuse and Information line (SAIL), British Columbia, Canada

http://seniorsfirstbc.ca/programs/sail – Tel: 604 437 1940; (toll
free) 1866 437 1940 – Support and information line for seniors
about elder abuse

AUSTRALIA

Advance Care Planning Australia

www.advancecareplanning.org.au – Australian government
website about advance care planning

Aged Care Crisis

www.agedcarecrisis.com/resources/nursing-home-checklist#the
nursing home – Checklist from a consumer based advocacy
group

Alzheimer's Australia

www.fightdementia.org.au – Tel: 1800 100 500. Telephone
advisory service about dementia care

Carers Australia
www.carersaustralia.com.au – Tel: 1800 242 636. Telephone advisory service for caregivers

Choice
www.choice.com.au/health-and-body/healthy-ageing/ageing-and-retirement/articles/aged-care-guide – Information about choosing aged care from a consumer advocacy group

Dementia Support Australia
www.dementia.com.au – Tel: 1800 699 799 (24-hour helpline). Telephone advisory and referral service about dementia care

Department of Health
www.health.gov.au/internet/main/publishing.nsf/content/acp – Australian government website with information and links about advance care planning, for consumers and health professionals

Elder Abuse Prevention Unit
www.eapu.com.au – Elder abuse telephone helpline. Tel: 1300 651 192 or 07 3867 2525. A charity-run helpline and information service to support older people

Feros Care
www.feroscare.com.au/?s=checklist+choosing+right+aged+care – Checklist about choosing aged care from a not-for-profit provider

Lifeline
www.lifeline.org.au – Tel: 13 11 14. 24-hour crisis line for mental health, including suicide issues

My Aged Care

www.myagedcare.gov.au/considering-aged-care-home/finding-aged-care-home – Information about aged care from the federal government

www.myagedcare.gov.au/considering-aged-care-home/preparing-move – Information about aged care from the federal government

www.myagedcare.gov.au/legal-information/elder-abuse-concerns – Information and support contact details for each Australian state and territory
www.myagedcare.gov.au – Tel: 1800 200 422. Telephone advisory service

National Association of Loss and Grief (NALAG)

www.nalag.org.au – Tel: +612 6882 9222. Telephone and website service about grief

NSW Elder Abuse Helpline

www.elderabusehelpline.com.au – Tel: 1800 628 221

Office of the Public Advocate Victoria

www.publicadvocate.vic.gov.au

Palliative Care Australia

http://palliativecare.org.au/support-and-services/advance-care-planning – Website about support and services regarding advance care planning, including a helpful 'how to' guide and contact details for each state.

Seniors Rights Victoria

https://seniorsrights.org.au – Tel: 1300 368 821. Telephone support and advice services

NEW ZEALAND

Age Concern
www.ageconcern.org.nz/ACNZPublic/Services/EANP/ACNZ_
Public/Elder_Abuse_and_Neglect.aspx – Tel: 0800 32 668 65.
Free and professional confidential helpline and information
website

Alzheimers New Zealand
www.alzheimers.org.nz/about-dementia/booklets-and-fact-
sheets – Booklets and factsheets

Eldernet
www.eldernet.co.nz/IM_Custom/ContentStore/Assets/9/0/2014
EN Checklist Residential Care.pdf – Checklist for choosing
residential care

Find a Rest Home
https://findaresthome.co.nz – Information about finding a rest
home

Ministry of Health
Tel: 0800 855 066 – For general enquiries about advance care
planning

Tel: 0800 611 116 – Free health advice information service

National Advance Care Planning Cooperative
www.advancecareplanning.org.nz and www.
advancecareplanning.org.nz/healthcare/resources/#tab_tab1 –
Resources and information, including advance care planning
forms and a 'how to' guide to advance care planning

ALTERNATIVE TERMS

Alternative terms	We have used
Aged care home, care home, nursing home, residential aged care, facility, residence	Care home
Proxy, substitute decision maker, durable or lasting or medical enduring power of attorney	Substitute decision maker
Older person, older adult, senior citizen, elder, older people, elderly	Older person, older people
Health and social care	UK only, health and social care
Your country, county, province, state, local government area	Your local area
Family doctor, GP, general practitioner, family physician, primary care physician	Family doctor
Family, friends, relatives	Family

REFERENCES

Alzheimer's Australia (2015) Information for family and friends. Help Sheet Number 4. Available at: https://www.fightdementia.org.au/files/helpsheets/Helpsheet-AboutDementia04-Information ForFamilyAndFriends_english.pdf, accessed 8 September 2017.

Alzheimer's Disease International (2012) *World Alzheimer Report 2012. Overcoming the Stigma of Dementia.* London: Alzheimer's Disease International.

American Psychological Association (2017) What is resilience? Available at: www.apa.org/helpcenter/road-resilience.aspx, accessed on 8 September 2017.

Aminzadeh, F., Dalziel, W.B., Molnar, F.J. and Garcia, L.J. (2009). 'Symbolic meaning of relocation to a residential care facility for persons with dementia.' *Aging and Mental Health,* 13(3), 487–496.

Australian Bureau of Statistics (2017) Australia's population by country of birth. Migration, Australia cat. no. 3412.0.

Australian Department of Health and Ageing (2011) Technical paper on the changing dynamics of residential aged care, prepared to assist the Productivity Commission Inquiry Caring for Older Australians. Australian Department of Health and Ageing, April 2011. Available at: www.pc.gov.au, accessed 21 June 2017.

Australian Institute of Health and Welfare (2012) Residential aged care in Australia 2010–11: a statistical overview. Aged care statistics series no. 36. Cat. No. AGE 68. Canberra: AIHW.

Australian Institute of Health and Welfare (2017) Characteristics of people in aged care. Available at: www.aihw.gov.au/aged-care/residential-and-home-care-2014-15/characteristics, accessed 20 March 2017.

Bailly, N., Joulain, M., Herve, C. and Alaphilippe, D. (2012) 'Coping with negative life events in old age: the role of tenacious goal pursuit and flexible goal adjustment.' *Aging and Mental Health,* 16, 431–437.

Bauer, M., McAuliffe, L., and Nay, R. (2007). 'Sexuality, health care and the older person: an overview of the literature.' *International Journal of Older People* 2(1), 63–68.

Bauer, M., Fetherstonhaugh, D., Tarzia, L., Nay, R. and Beattie, E. (2014) 'Supporting residents' expression of sexuality: the initial construction of a sexuality assessment tool for residential aged care facilities.' *BMC Geriatrics,* 14, 82–82.

Brown, J. (2012) 'The most difficult decision: dementia and the move into residential aged care.' Alzheimer's Australia NSW. Discussion paper no. 5.

Brownfield, L. (2017) Life with meaning – what makes us 'happy to be alive'. Presentation to Better Practice Conference Melbourne 2017.

Brownie, S., Horstmanshof, L. and Garbutt, R. (2014) 'Factors that impact residents' transition and psychological adjustment to long-term aged care: a systematic literature review.' *International Journal of Nursing Studies,* 51, 1654–1666.

Caffrey, C., Sengupta, M., Park-Lee, E., Moss, A., Rosenoff, E. and Harris-Kojetin, H. (2012) 'Residents living in residential care facilities: United States, 2010.' NCHS data brief, no 91. Hyattsville, MD: National Center for Health Statistics.

Cheston, R., Hancock, J. and White, P. (2016) 'A cross sectional investigation of public attitudes toward dementia in Bristol and South Gloucestershire using the approaches to dementia questionnaire.' *International Psychogeriatrics*, 28, 1717–1724.

Dow, B., Haralambous, B., Bremner, F. and Fearn, M. (2006) *What is Person-centred Care? A Literature Review.* Prepared by National Ageing Research Institute, February. Victorian Government Department of Human Services, Melbourne.

Doyle, C. and Roberts, G. (2016a) Human and civil rights of older people. *Encyclopedia of Geropsychology.* Berlin/Heidelberg, Germany: Springer Science, doi: 10.1007/978-981-287-080-3_291-1.

Doyle, C. and Roberts, G. (2016b) *A Review of Progress in the Development of Dementia Services at BlueCross.* Final report prepared for BlueCross. Melbourne: Australian Catholic University.

Ellis, J.M. (2010) 'Psychological transition in a residential care facility: older people's experiences.' *Journal of Advanced Nursing*, 66(5), 1159–1168.

Enz, K.F., Pillemer, D.B. and Johnson, K.M. (2016) 'The relocation bump: memories of middle adulthood are organized around residential moves.' *Journal of Experimental Psychology: General*, 145(8), 935–940.

Eriksson, H. and Sandberg, J. (2008) 'Transitions in men's caring identities: experiences from home-based care to nursing home placement.' *International Journal of Older People Nursing*, 3(2), 131–137.

Feil, N. (1993) *The Validation Breakthrough: Simple Techniques for Communicating with People with 'Alzheimer's-type Dementia.'* Baltimore, MD: Health Professions Press.

Fisher, J.M. (2000) Creating the Future? In J.W. Scheer (ed.) *The Person in Society: Challenges to a Constructivist Theory.* Giessen, Germany: Giessen Psychosozial-Verlag, pp.428–437.

Fisher, J.M. (2012) Fisher's process of personal change – revised 2012. Available at: www.businessballs.com/personalchangeprocess.htm, accessed 16 July 2017.

Forder, J. and Fernandez, J-L. (2011) *Length of Stay in Care Homes.* A report commissioned by Bupa. PSSRU Discussion Paper 2769. Canterbury: PSSRU.

Freedman, V.A. and Spillman, B.C. (2014) 'The residential continuum from home to nursing home: size, characteristics and unmet needs of older adults.' *Journals of Gerontology, Series B: Psychological Sciences and Social Sciences,* 69(7), S42–S50, doi: 10.1093/geronb/gbu120.

Gould. O.N., Dupuis-Blanchard, S., Villalon, L., Simard, M. and Ethier, S. (2015) 'Hoping for the best or planning for the future: decision making and future care needs.' *Journal of Applied Gerontology,* 36(8), 953–970.

Hardy, S.E., Concato, J. and Gill, T.M. (2002) 'Stressful life events among community-living older persons.' *Journal of General Internal Medicine,* 17, 841–847.

HelpAge International (2010a) Strengthening older people's rights: towards a UN convention. A resource for promoting dialogue on creating a new UN Convention on the rights of older persons. London: HelpAge International.

HelpAge International (2010b) Age helps. International human rights law and older people. London: HelpAge International.

HelpGuide (2017) Coping with grief and loss. Available at: www.helpguide.org/articles/grief/coping-with-grief-and-loss.htm, accessed 8 September 2017.

Heppenstall, C.P., Keeling, S., Hanger, H.C. and Wilkinson, T.J. (2014) 'Perceived factors which shape decision-making around the time of residential care admission in older adults: QA qualitative study.' *Australasian Journal on Ageing*, 33(1), 9–13.

Johnson, R.A. and Bibbo, J. (2014) 'Relocation decisions and constructing the meaning of home: a phenomenological study of the transition into a nursing home.' *Journal of Aging Studies*, 30, 56–63.

Katz, J.S. and Peace, S. (eds) (2003) *End of Life in Care Homes: a Palliative Care Approach*. Oxford, UK: Oxford University Press.

Ke, L.-S., Huang, X., Hu, W.-Y., O'Connor, M. and Lee, S. (2017) 'Experiences and perspectives of older people regarding advance care planning: a metasynthesis of qualitative studies.' *Palliative Medicine*, 31(5), 394–405.

Kelly, A., Conell-Price, J., Covinsky, K., Stijacic, I. *et al.* (2010) 'Lengths of stay for older adults residing in nursing homes at the end of life.' *Journal of the American Geriatrics Society*, 58, 1701–1706.

Kessing, L.V., Agerbo, E. and Mortensen, P.B. (2003) 'Does the impact of major stressful life events on the risk of developing depression change throughout life?' *Psychological Medicine*, 33(7), 1177–1184.

Koppitz, A.L., Dreizler, J., Altherr, J., Bosshard, G., Naef, R. and Imhof, L. (2017) 'Relocation experiences with unplanned admission to a nursing home: a qualitative study.' *International Psychogeriatrics*, 29(3), 517–527.

Kubler-Ross, E. (2005) *On Grief and Grieving: Finding the Meaning of Grief through the Five Stages of Loss*. London: Simon & Schuster Ltd.

Mahieu, L. and Gastmans, C. (2015) 'Older residents' perspectives on aged sexuality in institutionalized elderly care: a systematic literature review.' *International Journal of Nursing Studies,* 52(12), 1891–1905.

Manion, P.S. and Rantz, M.J. (1995) 'Relocation stress syndrome: a comprehensive plan for long-term care admissions: the relocation stress syndrome diagnosis helps nurses identify patients at risk.' *Geriatric Nursing,* 16, 108–112.

McCormick, W.C., Uomoto, J., Young, H., Graves, A.B. *et al.* (1996) 'Attitudes toward use of nursing homes and home care in older Japanese-Americans.' *Journal of the American Geriatrics Society,* 44(7), 769–777.

McGlade, C., Daly, E., McCarthy, J., Cornally, N. *et al.* (2017) 'Challenges in implementing an advance care planning programme in long-term care.' *Nursing Ethics,* 24(1), 87–99.

Meaningful Ageing Australia (2016) National guidelines for spiritual care in aged care. Melbourne: Meaningful Ageing Australia. Available at: https://meaningfulageing.org.au/wp-content/uploads/2016/08/National-Guidelines-for-Spiritual-Care-in-Aged-Care-DIGITAL.pdf, accessed 8 September 2017.

Medical Treatment Act 1988 (VIC) Available at: www.austlii.edu.au/au/legis/vic/consol_act/mta1988168, accessed 15 July 2017.

Mehrabian, A. (1981) *Silent Messages: Implicit Communication of Emotions and Attitudes.* Belmont, CA: Wadsworth.

Mignani, V., Ingravallo, F., Mariani, E. and Chattat, R. (2017) 'Perspectives of older people living in long-term care facilities and of their family members toward advance care planning discussions: a systematic review and thematic analysis.' *Clinical Interventions in Aging,* 12, 475–484.

Neher, J.O. (2004) *Like a River.* The Hastings Center Report 34.2 March/April.

Niebuhr, R. (1986) *The Essential Reinhold Niebuhr: Selected Essays and Addresses.* Newhaven, CT and London: Yale University Press. Edited by R. McAfee Brown.

Office for National Statistics (2013) What does the 2011 census tell us about older people. Available at: www.ons.gov.uk/peoplepopulationandcommunity/birthsdeathsandmarriages/ageing/articles/whatdoesthe2011censustellusaboutolderpeople/2013-09-06, accessed 16 July 2017.

Office for National Statistics (2014) Changes in the older resident care home population between 2001 and 2011. Available at: www.ons.gov.uk, accessed 20 March 2017.

Oren, S., Willerton, C. and Small, J. (2014) 'Effects of spaced retrieval training on semantic memory in Alzheimer's disease: a systematic review.' *Journal of Speech, Language and Hearing Research,* 57, 247–270.

Palliative Care Australia (2017) Understanding grief. Available at: www.Palliativecare.org.au, accessed 15 June 2017.

Peace (2003) 'The Development of Residential and Nursing Home Care in the United Kingdom.' In J.S. Katz and S. Peace (eds) *End of Life in Care Homes: A Palliative Care Approach.* Oxford, UK: Oxford University Press, pp.15–43.

Prince, D. and Butler, D. (2007) *Clarity Final Report: Aging in Place in America.* Nashville, TN: Prince Market Research.

Robinson A.L., Dickinson C., and Rousseau N. (2012) 'A systematic review of the effectiveness of advance care planning interventions for people with cognitive impairment and dementia.' *Age and Ageing* 41, 263–269.

Ronalds, C. (1989) *Residents' Rights in Nursing Homes and Hostels: Final Report.* Canberra: Australia Government Public Service.

Rubio, L., Dumitrache, C., Cordon-Pozo, E. and Rubio-Herrera, R. (2016) 'Coping; impact of gender and stressful life events in middle and in old age.' *Clinical Gerontologist* 39(5), 468–488.

Shalowitz, D.I., Garrett-Mayer, E. and Wendler, D. (2006) 'The accuracy of surrogate decision makers: a systematic review.' *Archives of Internal Medicine,* 166, 493–497.

Sone, T., Nakaya, N., Ohmori, K., Shimazu, T. *et al.* (2008) 'Sense of life worth living (Ikigai) and mortality in Japan: Ohsaki study.' *Psychosomatic Medicine,* 70, 709–715.

Statistics Canada (2017) Dwellings in Canada: Census of population, 2016. Cat. No. 98-200-X2016005. Ministry of Industry: Canada.

Thomas, K. and Lobo, B. (eds) (2011) *Advance Care Planning in End of Life Care.* New York: Oxford University Press.

United Nations General Assembly (1987) *UN convention against Torture and Other Cruel, Inhumane or Degrading Treatment of Punishment.* New York: UN.

Villar, F., Serrat, R., Faba, J. and Celdran, M. (2015) 'Staff reactions toward lesbian, gay, or bisexual (LGB) people living in residential aged care facilities (RACFs) who actively disclose their sexual orientation.' *Journal of Homosexuality,* 62(8), 1126–1143.

Xiao, L.D., Willis, E., Harrington, A., Gillham, D. *et al.* (2017) 'Resident and family member perceptions of cultural diversity in aged care homes.' *Nursing and Health Sciences,* 19(1), 59–65.

Yeboah, C.A. (2015) 'Choosing to live in a nursing home: a culturally and linguistically diverse perspective.' *Australian Journal of Primary Care,* 21, 239–244.

INDEX

Colleen Doyle is a research psychologist in Melbourne, Australia, with a PhD from The University of Adelaide, South Australia. She has worked in the UK, USA and Australia focusing on aged care and health service evaluation throughout her career, and has published a wide range of academic and technical evaluations including in the areas of dementia, mental health, chronic obstructive pulmonary disease and health policy. She has been the recipient of a Gerontological Society of America summer fellowship and an Alzheimer's Australia travelling fellowship and is currently an honorary professorial fellow at the Australian National Ageing Research Institute and Florey Institute of Neuroscience and Mental Health. She is national convenor and founder of the Psychology and Aging Interest Group in the Australian Psychological Society.

Gail Roberts is a registered nurse and social scientist. Gail has conducted research for the Victorian Parliament, private organisations and for Australian universities including ANU, La Trobe, Deakin, Melbourne and ACU. She has extensive experience in tertiary settings and in professional education, and has worked for state and federal government on public policy development, implementation and evaluation, and in advance care planning, aged care, population health and general practice. Her research interests are in dementia care, advance care planning, community care and the intersection between health, law and ethics in aged care.